*Advocacy Strategies
for
Health and Mental Health
Professionals*

Stuart L. Lustig, MD, MPH, is a medical director for Cigna Corporation. He is an adjunct associate professor of clinical psychiatry and until recently the director of psychiatric training in the Division of Child and Adolescent Psychiatry at the University of California, San Francisco School of Medicine. His clinical and research work involves advocacy for immigrants, refugees, and survivors of torture. He is an asylum network evaluator for Physicians for Human Rights and a human rights clinic trainer and evaluator for HealthRight International. He was a guest lecturer in the UCSF Medicine Law Collaborative, where he taught interdisciplinary approaches to advocacy and where he oversees the child psychiatry rotation for medical students, nurse practitioner students, and psychiatry residents. He has been a guest lecturer at the University of California Hastings College of the Law, where he offers refugee clinic seminars. Dr. Lustig developed a collaborative relationship between the child and adolescent psychiatry residency program and the San Francisco County Department of Public Health, where child psychiatry residents now rotate as part of their training in public-sector child psychiatry. Additionally, he developed an innovative curriculum on advocacy for first-year child psychiatry residents. He has authored numerous book chapters and scholarly journal articles.

Advocacy Strategies for Health and Mental Health Professionals

From Patients to Policies

Stuart L. Lustig, MD, MPH

EDITOR

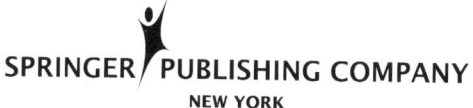

SPRINGER PUBLISHING COMPANY
NEW YORK

Copyright © 2012 Springer Publishing Company, LLC

All rights reserved.

No part of this publication may be reproduced, stored in a retrieval system, or transmitted in any form or by any means, electronic, mechanical, photocopying, recording, or otherwise, without the prior permission of Springer Publishing Company, LLC, or authorization through payment of the appropriate fees to the Copyright Clearance Center, Inc., 222 Rosewood Drive, Danvers, MA 01923, 978-750-8400, fax 978-646-8600, info@copyright.com or on the Web at www.copyright.com.

Springer Publishing Company, LLC
11 West 42nd Street
New York, NY 10036
www.springerpub.com

Acquisitions Editor: Sheri W. Sussman
Associate Editor: Kathryn Corasaniti
Composition: Newgen

ISBN: 978-0-8261-0906-4
E-book ISBN: 978-0-8261-0907-1

12 13 14/ 5 4 3 2 1

The author and the publisher of this Work have made every effort to use sources believed to be reliable to provide information that is accurate and compatible with the standards generally accepted at the time of publication. The author and publisher shall not be liable for any special, consequential, or exemplary damages resulting, in whole or in part, from the readers' use of, or reliance on, the information contained in this book. The publisher has no responsibility for the persistence or accuracy of URLs for external or third-party Internet websites referred to in this publication and does not guarantee that any content on such websites is, or will remain, accurate or appropriate.

Library of Congress Cataloging-in-Publication Data

Advocacy strategies for health and mental health professionals : from patients to policies / [edited by] Stuart L. Lustig.
   p. ; cm.
Includes bibliographical references and index.
ISBN 978-0-8261-0906-4 — ISBN 978-0-8261-0907-1 (E-book)
I. Lustig, Stuart L.
[DNLM: 1. Patient Advocacy—United States. 2. Lobbying—United States. 3. Patient Rights—United States. W 85.4]

362.1—dc23

2012016464

Special discounts on bulk quantities of our books are available to corporations, professional associations, pharmaceutical companies, health care organizations, and other qualifying groups.

If you are interested in a custom book, including chapters from more than one of our titles, we can provide that service as well.

For details, please contact:
Special Sales Department, Springer Publishing Company, LLC
11 West 42nd Street, 15th Floor, New York, NY 10036–8002
Phone: 877-687-7476 or 212-431-4370; Fax: 212-941-7842
Email: sales@springerpub.com

Printed in the United States of America by Gasch Printing.

To everyone who toils for a brighter tomorrow.

Contents

Contributors *xiii*
Foreword *xvii*
Preface *xxi*
Acknowledgments *xxv*

1. **Discovering Your Inner Advocate**   *1*
   Molly Lubin and Stuart L. Lustig
   The Importance of Advocacy   *1*
   Idealism and Advocacy   *3*
   Promoting Advocacy From Within and From Outside the Health Professions   *6*
   What You Bring to the Table, and Will Take From This Book   *9*
   Reflection Questions   *10*
   Practice Makes Perfect   *10*
   References   *10*

2. **Learning How to Advocate: Perspectives From Medical Educators**   *13*
   John Q. Young, Fumi Mitsuishi, and Lowell Tong
   The Advocacy Imperative   *13*
   The Advocacy Skills Gap   *15*
   What Needs to Be Learned?   *16*
   Educational Strategies That Do Not Work   *17*
   Educational Strategies That Work   *19*
   Putting Learning Principles Into Practice   *21*
   Case Study: The Institute for Healthcare Improvement   *24*
   Conclusion   *25*
   Reflection Questions   *25*
   Practice Makes Perfect   *25*
   References   *26*

3. Overview of the Political Advocacy Process   29
Richard L. Barnes
What Is Policy Advocacy?   29
Evaluating the Challenges to the Public Health Goal   31
An Alliance of Supporting Organizations   32
Evidence-Based Policy Design   34
The Strategic Plan   39
Executing the Strategic Plan   41
Policy Implementation and Evaluation   45
Reflection Questions   45
Practice Makes Perfect   45
References   46

4. Legislative Advocacy: Putting Your House in Order   51
Kristin Kroeger Ptakowski
How a Bill Becomes a Law   52
Advancing Your Cause   56
How to Communicate Your Message   57
Using the Media for Legislative Advocacy   60
Case Study: Reauthorization of the SCHIP Program   61
Reflection Questions   63
Practice Makes Perfect   63
References   63

5. How to Work With the Media   65
Aaron Levin
The Media Today   66
How Do I Start?   67
Crafting the Message   68
Earned Media Versus Paid Media   68
Get to Know Your Media   69
Contact List   70
Preparing for Interviews   71
Interview Basics   72
Avoid Jargon and Acronyms   72
Interviews and Television   73
Letters to the Editor   73
Op-Eds   74
Media Opportunities   75
Share Your Success   76
The Digital Realm   76
Social Media   76
Final Thoughts   78
Case Study: Healthy Minds, Healthy Lives   78
Reflection Questions   79
Practice Makes Perfect   79
References   79

6. **Is There a Lawyer in the House? When to Work With an Attorney** *81*
   Sarah S. Wessels and Megan Sandel
   Identifying Unmet Legal Needs *82*
   Case Study: Food and Utilities *84*
   Case Study: Eviction Defense *86*
   Case Study: Mice Are Threats to Health *87*
   Case Study: Special Needs for Child With Cerebral Palsy *88*
   Case Study: Disability Benefit Denials *90*
   How to Refer Patients to Legal Help *93*
   Medical–Legal Partnerships: A Model for Success *97*
   From Patients to Policies—Advocating for System Changes *99*
   Reflection Questions *102*
   Practice Makes Perfect *102*
   Notes *102*

7. **Class Action for Health Professionals** *105*
   Bruce L. Simon and Thomas K. Boardman
   Class Action Versus Individual Action *106*
   How Does a Class Action Work, Exactly? *107*
   Case Study: *Klay V. Humana, Inc.*, 382 F.3d 1241, 1274 (11th Cir. 2004) *115*
   Conclusion *119*
   Reflection Questions *119*
   Practice Makes Perfect *120*
   References *120*

8. **Leveraging Research Findings: Learning the Practice of Advocacy** *121*
   Geri L. Dickson
   Why Do Research? *122*
   Identifying the Right Problem *123*
   What Is Going to Be Big News? *125*
   Asking the Right Question(s) *127*
   Selecting the Right Analytic Method *129*
   Summarizing Findings *130*
   Case Study: A Qualitative Method Study of School Counselors *132*
   Case Study: Research Findings Used to Advocate for Expanding the Nursing Workforce *134*
   Lessons Learned From Using Research Findings in Health Care Advocacy *138*
   Conclusion *139*
   Reflection Questions *139*
   Practice Makes Perfect *139*
   References *140*

9. Working With Families and Community Organizations   143
Robert Hendren and Lee Grossman

Parent/Family Organizations as Partners—Why Do They
Form?   *144*
Case Study: Formation of the Autism Society of America   *145*
How Does the Health Professional Fit In?   *146*
How to Identify and Approach a Community Organization   *147*
Case Study: Bill of Rights for Children With Mental Health Disorders
and Their Families   *148*
Case Study: Autism Society of America Revisited   *150*
Case Study: Formation of the MIND Institute at the University Of
California, Davis   *152*
Case Study: My Son With Autism—An Advocacy Odyssey and
Message For Health Professionals (by Lee Grossman)   *153*
Reflection Questions   *155*
Practice Makes Perfect   *155*
References   *156*

10. Finding Funds   157
Tracy Mills

Funding Sources   *157*
Fundraising Roles and Responsibilities   *159*
Fundraising From Individuals   *161*
Case Study: Cultivating a Relationship   *166*
Case Study: The Importance of Connections   *167*
Case Study: The Importance of Focusing on the Donor   *169*
Case Study: Remember to Continue Communicating
With Donors   *171*
Volunteers   *172*
Case Study: Keeping Donors Involved With Your Cause   *173*
Final Points to Remember About Private Donors   *173*
Foundations and Corporations   *175*
Conclusion—The Results of Philanthropy   *178*
Reflection Questions   *178*
Practice Makes Perfect   *178*
References   *179*

11. A Comprehensive Strategy: Putting It All Together   181
Richard L. Barnes

The Problem   *182*
Finding Partners: A Coalition Is Reborn   *182*
Forging New, Powerful Partnerships   *183*
Leveraging Progress: On to the Legislature   *185*
From Legislators to Lawsuits   *187*
A Convergence of Strategies, a Fumble, and a Sprint to the
Finish   *188*
A Recap: Lessons Learned   *190*
Epilogue   *191*
References   *191*

Appendix

Introduction   *193*

Media Case Study

A Trio of Twitter Tales   *194*
Pierrette Mimi Poinsett

Research Case Study

Edgewood's Kinship Support Network: Using Research Findings to Develop a Community Program   *197*
Donald Cohon

Community Organizations Case Study

Partners in Health's Mental Health Program in Haiti: How an Initial Crisis Led to Advocacy for a Critical Unmet Need, an Expanded Program, Organizational Change, and a Shared National Mental Health Planning Effort   *202*
Giuseppe Raviola, Catherine Oswald, and Father Eddy Eustache

Index   *207*

Contributors

Richard L. Barnes, JD
Policy Researcher
Center for Tobacco Control Research and Education
University of California, San Francisco, CA

Thomas K. Boardman, JD
Founder
Hastings Science & Technology Law Journal
San Francisco, CA

Donald Cohon, PhD
Executive Vice President
Interdisciplinary Council on Developmental and Learning Disorders
Graduate School, Kentfield, CA

Geri L. Dickson, PhD, RN
Executive Director
New Jersey Collaborating Center for Nursing, Rutgers University, Newark, NJ

Father Eddy Eustache, MA
Zanmi Lasante/Partners in HealthCentral Plateau, Haiti

Lee Grossman, MS
President and CEO
Autism Society of America
Bethesda, MD

Robert Hendren, DO
Chief, Division of Child and Adolescent Psychiatry
Vice Chair, Department of Psychiatry
University of California, San Francisco School of Medicine
San Francisco, CA

Aaron Levin, MA
Senior Staff Writer
Psychiatric News
Arlington, VA

Molly Lubin, BA
Medical Student
University of California, San Francisco School of Medicine
San Francisco, CA

Stuart L. Lustig, MD, MPH
Medical Director, Cigna Corporation
Adjunct Associate Professor of Clinical Psychiatry
University of California, San Francisco School of Medicine
San Francisco, CA

Tracy Mills, BA
Director of Development
Department of Psychiatry
University of California, San Francisco School of Medicine
San Francisco, CA

Fumi Mitsuishi, MD, MS
Resident Physician
Department of Psychiatry
University of California, San Francisco
San Francisco, CA

Catherine Oswald, MPH
Zanmi Lasante/Partners in HealthCentral Plateau, Haiti

Pierrette Mimi Poinsett, MD
CEO Indigo Lotus Navigators, Petaluma, CA

Kristin Kroeger Ptakowski, BA
Senior Deputy Executive Director and Director
Government Affairs and Clinical Practice
American Academy of Child and Adolescent Psychiatry
Washington, DC

Giuseppe Raviola, MD
Department of Global Health and Social Medicine, Harvard Medical School
Department of Psychiatry, Children's Hospital Boston, and Harvard Medical School Partners in Health, Boston, MA

Megan Sandel, MD, MPH
National Medical Director
National Center for Medical-Legal Partnership
Director of Pediatric Healthcare for the Homeless at Boston Medical Center
Boston, MA

Bruce L. Simon, JD
Pearson, Simon, Warshaw & Penny, San Francisco and Los Angeles, CA

Lowell Tong, MD
Vice Chair for Education
Department of Psychiatry
University of California, San Francisco School of Medicine
San Francisco, CA

Sarah S. Wessels, JD
Director, JustHealth Foundation
Oakland, CA

John Q. Young, MD, MPA
Associate Director
Residency Training
University of California, San Francisco School of Medicine
San Francisco, CA

Foreword

The work goes on, the cause endures, the hope still lives and the dream shall never die. — Senator Edward M. Kennedy

Many years ago, my father was a state senator in Michigan. As a young boy, it was not unusual in our home to receive telephone calls from his constituents voicing their concerns about a specific issue and asking for "something to be done." Even today, I remember one caller very well. A man who lived on the next block would call my father every time it rained. He would complain about a large pool of water in the street directly in front of his home. During each call, my father listened attentively while expressing an understanding of the problem and empathy for the man's plight. After a series of these phone calls during one particularly rainy spring, I remember my father getting off the telephone and stating with some exasperation, "I need to get that darn [not his exact words] street fixed." The man called only one subsequent time and that was to thank my father for getting the street fixed. Thus, my introduction to advocacy.

Nearly 50 years later, I found myself living in Massachusetts where I experienced my own version of street flooding. Like many others in the state, I had become frustrated with poor access to mental health care and late identification of children with treatable psychiatric disorders, complex and fragmented "nonsystems" of care for children, overcrowded emergency rooms boarding children in need of intense psychiatric treatments, children stuck in costly inpatient units for weeks awaiting acceptance to more appropriate community-based care, lack of school and community-based services for want of sustainable funding, and poor integration of mental health with primary care clinicians (Greenberg, Darcy, & DeMaso, 2009). Needless to say, this was a bigger problem than water in front of my home and required a larger collective voice—the Children's Mental Health Campaign (referred to hereafter as "Campaign").

In 2006, a conversation between leaders from Children's Hospital Boston (CHB) and the Massachusetts Society for the Prevention of Cruelty to Children (MSPCC) led to a joint decision to initiate a campaign that would emphasize systemic approaches to addressing serious children's health issues and building partnerships with other organizations in advancing systemic change (Greenberg et al., 2009). The end goal was to reform the state's mental health system to ensure that all children with psychiatric disorders have access to coordinated and culturally appropriate prevention, early identification, and evidence-based treatment services.

We invited three organizations—Health Care for All, Health Law Advocates, and the Parent Professional Advocacy League—to form with us a core that would lead and direct the campaign. Recognizing the need for a much larger group of supporters to give the Campaign legitimacy, generate pressure on the state legislature, and build a financial base to sustain a long-term effort, the campaign did not "go public" until it had received the support of a critical mass of more than 30 key stakeholders: health care organizations representing providers, families, legal, and mental health advocates (Greenberg et al., 2009).

The Campaign formally began in November 2006 with a State House press conference, at which a policy paper "Children's Mental Health in the Commonwealth: The Time Is Now" was released (MSPCC & CHB, 2006). Coauthored by MSPCC and CHB, the paper described the children's mental health care system as "a complicated maze of fractured care, inadequate insurance coverage, programs too few and far between, and access defined by limitations in covered diagnoses and services," resulting in an estimated 100,000 children in Massachusetts not receiving needed mental health care. The report provided strong underlying support for the policy changes sought by the Campaign.

The Campaign soon grew into an active and diverse coalition of 135 organizations, representing providers, child and health care advocates, health policy experts, and educators, as well as countless families of children with mental illness. The Campaign was a carefully constructed initiative to include research and policy analysis, legislative drafting, coalition building, legislative engagement, fund raising, and media relations. The gradual expansion of the coalition built momentum and soon had a strong and visible presence in legislative districts throughout the state and in the corridors of the state house. The campaign also identified champions inside the Massachusetts legislature who played critical roles in educating and building strong support among their colleagues.

The efforts of the Campaign culminated with the signing of landmark legislation, Chapter 321 of the Acts of 2008, in a single 2-year legislative term (Commonwealth of Massachusetts, 2008). It marked a significant step in reaching our goals to (a) identify, diagnose, and treat mental health issues early in the life of children by promoting behavioral health screening and providing behavioral health consultations for children in early education and preschool settings; (b) provide schools with the tools necessary to identify children with behavioral health problems; (c) ensure that children receive care in the most appropriate and least restrictive settings; and (d) promote coordination between the multiple professionals and state agencies that interact with children with mental health needs. In a *Boston Globe* op-ed, former First Lady Rosalynn Carter remarked that this legislation laid the foundation for creating a "comprehensive and coordinated system of evidence-based mental health prevention, diagnosis, and treatment that is accessible to all children, adolescents, and families" (Carter, 2008). Now in its fourth year, the Campaign work has shifted to implementation of the legislation that in many ways has been less exciting, but by no means any less important.

So how did this happen? The timing was right. The mental health problems of children and the problematic child mental health care system had been well delineated in previous national white papers (President's New Freedom Commission on Mental Health, 2003; U.S. Department of Health and Human Services, 1999). In Massachusetts, a 2006 federal court ruling that the Commonwealth had violated the federal Medicaid Act by failing to provide appropriate home-based mental health care to an estimated 15,000 children provided a powerful impetus for creating an integrated child mental health care system. The election of a Democratic governor created a more favorable political climate, while passage of significant health care reform law positioned Massachusetts as a leader in health reform. The aforementioned "The Time Is Now" white paper laid out a cogent and implementable policy that could address the problems.

Policy change happens when there are clearly defined problems that are commonly understood, a cogent policy that addresses these needs, and a political climate that is receptive to the issue (Kingdon, 2003). There was also another critical variable that allowed change to occur—collaborators. The building of working partnerships was absolutely critical to the Campaign's success. The development of a unified coalition with providers, families, and legal and mental health advocates who could influence the legislative process was important. It takes the diverse knowledge, skills, persistence, dedication, and work of many individuals to advocate as successfully and on such a large scale as the Campaign.

But where does one learn to be an effective advocate? Where do health and mental health professionals learn the requisite skills and strategies? Unfortunately, up until now, they are generally not taught at all. When taught, the tedious task of identifying salient or seminal articles on advocacy combined with time pressures and/or incomplete searches result in it not being done well. With the publication of this textbook, those days are gone! This comprehensive book incorporates the expertise of national authorities into a pragmatic and useful format that begins by helping the reader understand his or her own individual motivations regarding advocacy and ends with the reader being able to "put it all together." This book is truly a welcome alternative to the teaching of the past.

Today, I am sure that the street in front of the man's house remains dry. He knew the work that needed to be done and never gave up in his effort to see it happen. Just as his street needed repair, so our health care system needs attention. This textbook provides the advocacy strategies that are critically needed to remedy the problems. The time is still now; let's go to work.

David R. DeMaso, MD
Psychiatrist-in-Chief and Chairman of Psychiatry
The Leon Eisenberg Chair in Psychiatry
Children's Hospital Boston
Professor of Psychiatry and Pediatrics
Harvard Medical School

REFERENCES

Carter, R. (2008, July 10). A leap in mental care for children. *Boston Globe.*

Greenberg, J., Darcy, K., & DeMaso, D. R. (2009). Advocating children's mental health care. *Children's Hospital Today, Spring,* 16–19.

Kingdon, J. W. (2003). *Agendas, alternatives and public policies* (2nd ed.). New Jersey: Longman Classics in Political Science.

Massachusetts Society for the Prevention of Cruelty to Children & Children's Hospital Boston. *Children's Mental Health in the Commonwealth: The Time Is Now,* November 2006, online: www.mspcc.org/document.doc?id=167

The 187th General Court of the Commonwealth of Massachusetts. Session Law Chapter 321, *An Act Relative to Children's Mental Health.* August 20, 2008, online: www.malegislature.gov/Laws/SessionLaws/Acts/2008/Chapter321

The President's New Freedom Commission on Mental Health. *Achieving the Promise: Transforming Mental Health Care in America, Executive Summary,* July 2003, online: http://govinfo.library.unt.edu/mentalhealthcommission/reports/FinalReport/toc_exec.html

U.S. Department of Health and Human Services. (1999). *Mental Health: A Report of the Surgeon General—Executive Summary.* Rockville, MD: U.S. Department of Health and Human Services, Substance Abuse and Mental Health Services Administration, Center for Mental Health Services, National Institutes of Health, National Institute of Mental Health.

Preface

Congratulations! We assume you picked up this book, and maybe even have already purchased it, because you realize that innovation and change in health care depend upon individuals like you who are strongly motivated to make the world a healthier place for everyone. That said, you have intuited that your knowledge of disease and well-being, obtained from your vantage point in medicine, nursing, pharmacy, dentistry, psychology, public health, or another field, has not been sufficient to help you achieve your vision. Perhaps you know what additional tools you need. Maybe you are not quite sure what is lacking but sense that you need some additional skills, and that you must partner with some other allies.

I decided to put together this volume because I wish I had had one just like it when I began my advocacy work on behalf of refugees seeking political asylum. A few of the lessons contained here I learned the hard way, along my own advocacy path. Most of the material in this book, however, I never learned until I read what the contributing authors had to say.

Although over the past decade multiple books were written to guide health care professionals in their advocacy work, none are specifically for health professionals as a unified constituency inclusive of all disciplines and stages of training. Some books target subpopulations of health and allied health care workers, such as nurses or clinical psychologists. Others place health care professionals within a larger continuum of those who work toward social justice in some capacity. Still others list health care professionals as a primary audience, but with an exclusionary focus on a specific issue such as tobacco policy or care of the elderly. This volume fills a void by providing a comprehensive summary of advocacy techniques appropriate for multiple topic areas, geared toward health professionals in all disciplines and at various levels of training and expertise. And so we begin.

Chapter 1, "Discovering Your Inner Advocate," reviews the importance of health advocacy and the state of idealism and exhorts you to do an inventory of your own motivations and strengths that you bring to the table.

A unique contribution of this book is the next chapter, Chapter 2, "Learning How to Advocate: Perspectives From Medical Educators." Health educators explain, based on adult learning theory, how to learn the material in this volume and how targets of advocacy, who are also adult learners, receive what advocates want to teach.

Chapter 3, "Overview of the Political Advocacy Process," written by an attorney-turned-lobbyist, is followed by a thorough but understandable description of the legislative process in Chapter 4, "Legislative Advocacy: Putting Your House in Order," written by a legislative affairs director for a major medical association. Chapter 5, "How to Work With the Media," written by a professional medical reporter, offers the health professional step-by-step approaches for utilizing various forms of media, whether print, television, or online, to advance advocacy issues.

We next address legal aspects of advocacy in Chapters 6 and 7. The first of these ("Is There a Lawyer in the House? When to Work With an Attorney") describes how health professionals can partner with attorneys for case-based advocacy. This chapter, coauthored by a physician and an attorney, covers a range of issues where medical and legal input can advance the health of patients. The next chapter, "Class Action for Health Professionals," written by two attorneys with extensive experience in class-action lawsuits in the health arena, discusses litigation as an advocacy tool that health professionals can leverage to further their goals.

Additional, seldom-covered topics appear in the remainder of the book. Chapter 8, "Leveraging Research Findings: Learning the Practice of Advocacy," has particular relevance for health professionals, most of whom have received basic training in research techniques. In this chapter, a nurse researcher discusses key aspects of designing research studies and disseminating the findings, learning the practice of advocacy, for maximal traction in a policy area. Chapter 9, "Working With Families and Community Organizations," is written by a mental health professional with experience in running a major family-funded institute. It reviews core concepts of working with family and community organizations as stakeholders in the advancement of common advocacy goals. Chapter 10, "Finding Funds," written by a major university's development officer, discusses strategies for funding these goals, whether through individuals, foundations, or corporations. Chapter 11, "A Comprehensive Strategy: Putting It All Together," uses a complex case study to highlight several of the strategies outlined in the book. In addition to the case study in Chapter 11, briefer case studies in all the chapters and in the Appendix showcase how specific skills and tactics come to life.

The field of health care has expanded vastly over the past century, as a consequence of social and economic change. Social and economic disadvantage contributes to poor health and disease. Health care professionals have collectively taken on new responsibilities, learned new skills, and extended their range of activities to include advocacy activities. We now routinely acknowledge the personal, social, and financial situations of our patients when planning treatment, but we can do better than merely noting the circumstances of our patients outside of the clinic. We can go far in eliminating both social and medical disparities by using our knowledge and influence to address social injustice and advocate for change. We hope this book will be your guide and your partner on this journey.

Stuart L. Lustig, MD, MPH

Acknowledgments

I owe a debt of gratitude to my students and trainees who, over the years, have inspired me with their own pursuits of a better world. In particular, I thank the child psychiatry trainees at the University of California, San Francisco, who have enthusiastically participated in our newly designed advocacy course on which this textbook was based and helped me better understand best practices for teachers and learners: Rajan Bahl, Farshid Farrahi, Alyse Han, Jefferson Joseph, Melissa Lorang, Erik Sandegard, Michael Swetye, and Shivani Verma. This book is intended for students of advocacy just like them. I thank my course codirector Basil Bernstein, a worthy advocate in his own right. I appreciate how Lynn Ponton, Jess Shatkin, and Laura Bergheim relentlessly encouraged me in this and other writing projects. Thanks to Robert Hendren for commenting on an early draft of this book's outline. My coauthor on the first chapter, Molly Lubin, with her resolute dedication to worthy causes, reminds us all of why there is hope for our planet. Meanwhile, all the authors of the chapters and case studies in this volume have been so accommodating of the publication schedule and the editing demands I have placed on them, all the while working to convey their important instructions for future advocates. I am grateful for the wisdom of Barry Gurdin, without whom I would not have found my way to Springer Publishing Company. I thank Springer's editor Jennifer Perillo for her vision of this book's potential; our conversations helped shape its direction and scope. I also thank Springer's editor Kathryn Corasaniti, whose constant guidance helped transform vision into reality, and the production team at Springer, especially Rose Mary Piscitelli, for ensuring that the reality would be optimal for all students of advocacy. Lastly, I am deeply grateful to my new wife, Haiyan Yang, who sacrificed so much to allow me the time and space I needed to achieve this goal.

1

Discovering Your Inner Advocate

MOLLY LUBIN AND STUART L. LUSTIG

A life without cause is a life without effect.—Dildano, in the movie *Barbarella*

THE IMPORTANCE OF ADVOCACY

The book you hold in your hands is the one many of us wish we had had when we were health care students and passionate about our reasons for choosing a life in the healing professions. These reasons are numerous: A burning desire to master and expand the science; a sense of gratitude or duty because of health care we or a relative received; a family tradition of healing; or perhaps a moral compass guided by social and health justice. But there is much to be done away from the bedside and outside the office or pharmacy, and a lot to know about how to change the world beyond the care of individual patients. This book covers a practical set of skills that augment the legitimacy of our professions in expanding the scope of our advocacy work. It aims to present advocacy work as a mainstay of health care, and is addressed to anyone who works in health care and those who would like to extend their voice and influence to address the social inequalities that adversely affect the health of their patients.

Health care in the United States today is the focus of impassioned debates and initiatives that galvanize millions of people. Doctors, nurses, dentists, and other health care professionals have been central to the struggle to eliminate health care disparities and to provide better health for all. By attending lobbying events, rallies, and press conferences, working with community organizations, and appealing to members of Congress, in addition to our clinical practice, we have taken leading roles in shaping a society that is most conducive to the physical and emotional health of its members. Indeed, social and political advocacy are essential activities of the health care professional.

Activism is not the work of lone visionaries; rather, national organizations of health care professionals avidly support the activist commitments of their members and drive their own initiatives. The American Medical Association (AMA) has sponsored community programs, partnered with local governments, published resource manuals, and lobbied and testified before Congress in support of public health measures ranging from violence prevention to obesity management to the elimination of health care disparities (AMA, n.d.). The American Dental Association (ADA) has also supported community health initiatives, most notably the fluoridation of drinking water, to which end it has worked with state and national governments and nongovernmental agencies (ADA, n.d.). Both the AMA and the American Nurse's Association (ANA) ardently backed the health care reform bill of 2010. The AMA spent $22 million toward passage of the bill (Vaida, 2011). The ANA website applauds the efforts of nurses nationwide and implores them to keep moving forward "The ink may have dried on healthcare reform,...[but]...our work is not done. We need YOU to stay active and involved!" (ANA, n.d.). This fighting spirit, then, is not one that should wax and wane depending on circumstances but, rather, should suffuse the ongoing work of the health care professional.

Health professionals can help their patients most profoundly and enduringly by engaging with their social and cultural milieus. The formation of medical–legal partnerships, which will be discussed in great detail in Chapter 6, is one example of how health care professionals can use their skills and knowledge outside of the clinic to further advance the health and welfare of their patients. Medical–legal partnerships serve a needed role in those situations in which, as the National Center for Medical-Legal Partnership (NCMLP) puts it, "medicine is not enough" (NCMLP). Through these unique collaborations that now operate at more than 235 health institutions nationwide, physicians and lawyers together can address "social determinants of health and seek to eliminate barriers to healthcare in order to help vulnerable populations meet their basic needs and stay healthy," advocating for services ranging from prevention of utility shut off during winter months to arranging for mold removal from homes of asthmatics (NCMLP). The success of these partnerships has been increasingly recognized and, indeed, the AMA recently released a newsletter article extolling the value of medical–legal partnerships, encouraging doctors to get involved (Sorrel, 2011).

IDEALISM AND ADVOCACY

A strong sense of idealism and commitment to social justice has often led nurses, physicians, and other health care professionals to their respective fields. This altruism has, in turn, inspired many to advocate tirelessly for the health and well-being of their patients outside of their clinic, as well as in traditional clinical settings. In this section we will first examine the meaning of idealism, especially the way in which it relates to health care and how it can foster advocacy work. We will then look at evidence for an alarming decline of idealism among health care professionals over the past half century, one that threatens to curb the type of activism and advocacy efforts in which so many have engaged.

As put forth by the Association of American Medical Colleges (AAMC), one of the most valued attributes of a physician is a work ethic rooted in idealism. The AAMC states that "embedded in the practice of medicine" are "the highest ethical principles" of "altruism, honesty, integrity, and the intention to help, comfort, and heal others " (AAMC, n.d., p. 6). This resonates with the Random House dictionary's definition of idealism as "the cherishing or pursuit of high or noble principles, purposes, [and] goals" (Random House Webster's College Dictionary, 1998). Medical educators in the University of Texas Medical School's Department of Family Medicine have further described idealism in medicine as the heartfelt desire to achieve "relief of suffering and improved quality of life for all humankind," by way of "volunteerism, service to under-served peoples, and concern for the health of society as a whole" (Smith & Weaver, 2006). That is, an idealistic physician carries out her work because she genuinely desires to mitigate suffering and help others, not simply because it is her job to perform this work.

Health professions attract idealists, just as the AAMC would hope. David Shaywitz and Dennis Ausiello of Harvard Medical School's Pasteur Center, a clinical research educational program, write that "concern for the health of others defines, above everything else, what it means to be a physician, and represents why so many of us were attracted to this calling" (Shaywitz & Ausiello, 2002). Training for a degree in medicine, nursing, dentistry, physical therapy, psychology, or in any other allied health profession is rigorous and exhausting. Those who choose to pursue these fields and remain committed in spite of the demands that come with that decision throughout an arduous training process are often highly motivated and determined to contribute to the health and well-being of society.

Clinical work that is driven by idealism may lead not only to more meaningful care of patients in the clinic, but to a sincere concern and genuine effort at providing for their health and well-being outside the clinic, as well. Physician and humanitarian Paul Farmer calls his idealism a motivating factor for the boundless acts of service that he has performed around the world. He describes "areas of moral clarity," that is, situations in which there is no option but to act, in hopes of alleviating or mitigating suffering (as cited in Kidder, 2003). Furthermore, as Shaywitz and Aussiello explain it, acts of service or voluntarism will help us gain an even fuller sense of our own idealism and of the values that our professions hold dear (Shaywitz & Ausiello, 2002). Thus, the relationship between idealism and service-oriented or advocacy work is mutually reinforcing.

Unfortunately, we can observe a decline of idealism in the health care professions today. Many commentators have pointed to structural factors in modern medicine and in medical education as the causes of growing cynicism and burnout. A 2002 article in the *Journal of the American Medical Association* (JAMA) described physician burnout as a syndrome including "emotional exhaustion, cynicism, and perceived clinical ineffectiveness, and a sense of depersonalization in relationships with coworkers, patients, or both," which arises in large part from overwork and insufficient time to care meaningfully for patients (Spickard, 2002). In 2007, CNN featured an account by a second-year medical student, Emily Breidbart, who describes the cumulative effect of time constraint and medical student debt: "We start out in medical school as idealists. We thirst for clinical experience. We want to explore all of our options, and help those who can't afford healthcare. But somewhere along the line, we start taking off our rose-colored glasses" (Breidbart, 2007). In 2010, the *New York Times* reported that top medical schools were questioning whether they had created doctors who "lack humanity, who see patients as diseases rather than as whole people, and who have what the medical literature calls 'ethical erosion'—a loss of idealism, empathy, morality" (Hartocollis, 2010). The article suggests that as medical students memorize hundreds of anatomical components and biochemical molecules, they may come to view their patients as merely agglomerates of these parts. This attitude, coupled with increasing workload and less time to build buoying relationships with patients, has the potential to chip away relentlessly at the motivation and selfless drive of young physicians.

Next, we will track the erosion of idealism that has occurred over the past half century as health care students have progressed through their careers. We can see that cynicism about both the practice of health care and patients has increasingly supplanted idealism, sapping clinicians of their motivation to advocate for the welfare of their patients outside the clinic.

The attitudes of health care professionals have been a cause for concern ever since they were first studied systematically in the 1950s. The first organized study of medical student attitudes, Becker and Geer's 1958 "The Fate of Idealism in Medical School," found that incoming medical students largely thought that "the practice of medicine...[was] a wonderful thing and that they...[were] going to devote their lives to service to mankind," but that they became less idealistic over the first 2 years of school (Becker & Geer, 1958). Their original drive and optimism for working with patients faded as they memorized long lists of facts for exams. In the third year, students were likely to view patients with chronic diseases as "creating extra work without extra compensation in knowledge." The authors noted that as students prepared for graduation, their original idealism reasserted itself. Nevertheless, the negativity and pessimism that many of these students experienced at various times in their schooling would certainly have some detrimental effect on their future careers.

Since the days of Becker and Geer's study, however, it has become only more difficult for medical students to retain the idealism they possess. A 1974 review of the literature on attitudes of medical students concluded that attitude was a serious problem and that medical schools should select students on the basis of their potential to maintain a positive attitude (Rezler, 1974). Fifteen years later, an additional study showed that medical students viewed themselves as becoming increasingly cynical and concerned with making money, warning that severe burnout and impairment could result (Wolf, 1989).

Studies from the past 20 years have shown that with every additional year of training, medical students grow increasingly negative and lacking in compassion. Unlike the medical students of Becker and Geer's study who recovered their idealism upon completion of medical school, today's students become even more cynical as time passes. One study of Kentucky medical students showed that as they progressed through their third year clerkships, they become less likely to believe that physicians love their jobs or that they themselves could make a difference in the well-being of their patients (Griffith & Wilson, 2001). A follow-up study by the same authors showed that throughout internship and residency, this pessimism only grows (Griffith & Wilson, 2003). Students increasingly come to believe that all elderly patients are hopelessly demented and that all patients who come in with complaints of pain are hoping to procure painkillers that they can sell or abuse. When physicians begin to believe their patients are unable to be helped or are immoral, the chance that these same physicians will seek to engage in advocacy or service work on their patients' behalf diminishes greatly. This sense of cynicism pervades the fictional account of a busy hospital service in *House of God*, in which physicians dehumanize their patients by means of disparaging categorizations which serve as a shorthand for clinical strategies. Almost as bad, the best care is no care; the interns learning medicine in their prestigious hospital quickly discover that committing acts of medical care only hurts their patients, rather than helps them (Shem, 1988).

Not only medical students and residents, but other types of health care professionals today also experience similar burnout and loss of faith in their professions. "The Lived Experience of Becoming an Occupational Therapist" describes the disillusionment that occupational therapists experience as they begin their practice and discover that the hopes and goals that they hold for their patients are often unrealistic (Tryssenaar, 1999). Meanwhile, a study of idealism and values among nurses noted the frustration inherent in the first 2 years of practice, as the reality of clinical work often fails to meet nurses' ideals and expectations (Maben, 2007). Taken as a whole, these studies and treatises indicate that this loss of optimism and disenchantment is widespread across many fields of health care professionals.

As educators in medicine, nursing, and other fields have become increasingly cognizant of this decline in idealism, they have become increasingly alarmed. Jill Maben of Britain's National Nursing Research Unit voices the direness of the situation by asking whether we should change the very mandate of nursing to make it more compatible with the attitudes of nurses (Maben, 2007). Many others in the field of health care have proposed various innovations and programs intended to boost the morale of students and early career professionals. We will now look at some recent initiatives to counter this erosion of idealism.

PROMOTING ADVOCACY FROM WITHIN AND FROM OUTSIDE THE HEALTH PROFESSIONS

For the past 10 years medical, dental, and nursing schools have made use of various strategies to increase students' desires to care for underserved populations and to advocate for the welfare of their patients outside of the clinic. Such initiatives include the formation of local and international community service electives as well as intensive mentorship and support programs. National policy organizations have recommended an increased focus on service-learning in health professional training and private foundations have begun to provide more funding to support the development of advocacy skills in students. In this section we will examine the objectives of these initiatives and the motivations that underlie their formation. It will become clear that health professional schools and those invested in their success have recognized the ongoing crisis of student burnout and apathy. These investors now prioritize the creation of a new generation of health care providers with a strong sense of community responsibility and commitment to social justice.

In recent years, medical training programs have offered students international medical electives with the hope that these experiences will attract them to working among diverse or underserved populations (Godkin, 2003). For example, from 1997 to 2005, educators at the University of Texas Medical Branch in Galveston provided 66 medical students with a 4-week elective course in rural Guatemala to help them become "socially responsible and idealistic" physicians. This elective was so successful in increasing its participants' "compassion, volunteerism, and interest in serving international populations" that faculty members recommended that international electives become a more central part of nationwide medical training (Smith & Weaver, 2006). Similarly, 21 resident surgeons at the University of California, Los Angeles participated in international surgical missions through Operation Smile. After these experiences, their self-reported newfound compassion, confidence, cultural sensitivity, sense of personal responsibility, and interest in volunteering among underserved populations were so encouraging that faculty members at this institution called for international surgical mission work to become a widespread part of the surgical residency training (Campbell, 2010). When medical schools and residency programs advocate for the addition of these international experiences to an already tightly packed curriculum, it becomes clear just how highly they prioritize the development of future leaders in community health.

Another way in which medical schools have expressed their growing commitment to bolstering students' interests in social justice and caring for the underserved is through instituting intensive faculty-sponsored mentorship and support systems for students who have taken an interest in this type of work (Wear & Kuczewski, 2008). One example that demonstrates well the institutionalization of such support structures is the University of California's "Program in Medical Education for Urban Under-Served," known as "PRIME-US." Launched in 2007, PRIME-US offers additional education in health disparities to a subset of medical students at several University of California medical schools. Its goal is to train a cohort of physicians who will be able to provide better care for California's most vulnerable and disadvantaged. A key component of this highly valued, state-funded program is its extensive student mentorship activities (Nation, Gerstenberger, & Bullard, 2007); indeed, the program's website states explicitly that the job of PRIME-US is to "support and sustain" the commitment of medical students to working among the urban underserved (PRIME-US; University of California School of Medicine). The formation of these support programs indicates the recognition by medical educators that simply exposing students to homeless or underserved populations is not enough; rather, they must also provide ongoing motivation and guidance that will empower students to transform a meaningful experience, such as working at a homeless clinic, into a lifelong career path.

Physician advocacy outside of the clinic is a priority of policy makers as well as educators. A 2003 report by a task force convened to investigate the future of the academic health center states that institutions of medical learning must produce physicians willing to serve indigent patients (The Commonwealth Fund, 2003). According to the report, students should spend time among geographically or financially underserved populations, faculty should role model their own work with the indigent, and schools should form partnerships with local communities. The 2010 report of the Liaison Committee on Medical Education, the national body that accredits medical schools, states that a medical school must provide an academic environment conducive to "service learning" (Liaison Committee on Medical Education, 2010), such as "a structured learning experience that combines community service with preparation and reflection." Furthermore, medical students thus engaged should "provide community service in response to community-identified concerns and learn about the context in which service is provided...and [about] their roles as citizens and professionals." To optimize service learning, the report suggests that schools could develop partnerships with local communities and offer public presentations and forums. This emphasis on service learning and social responsibility points, then, to a revised conception of a health professional school that not only trains students in the technical skills of medicine, dentistry, or nursing, but also inculcates them with a sense of civic responsibility and skills necessary for community engagement.

This trend is not limited to medical education; other types of health professional schools have initiated similar attempts to prepare students to work in disadvantaged communities and among patients with complex sociomedical needs. A study of seven dental schools in six states found that there was a widespread desire among dental educators and public health officials for dental education to become more responsive to public need (Davis, 2007). This sentiment is reflected in the fact that dental schools have in the past 5 years promoted service learning as a means of encouraging students' civic engagement and their interest in working in resource-poor settings (Aston-Brown, 2009; Hood, 2009). In 2005, dental students at the University of Missouri partnered with the Boys and Girls Club of Kansas City to provide free dental screenings to impoverished children. Students afterward reported a newfound enthusiasm for working in a public health setting (Aston-Brown, 2009). Another program at the University of Missouri placed dental hygiene students in community care settings for individuals with special needs, including those with complex medical problems and developmental disabilities. After completing the experience students were more interested in working with patients with disabilities, and had a greater awareness of the dental hygienist's capacity to provide service to a disadvantaged community (Keselyak, 2007).

Private foundations have also supported the involvement of students and young professionals in advocacy and social justice work. For example, the Albert Schweitzer Fellowship provides funding for selected community health projects of graduate students in the health and human services fields. This fellowship program was launched in 1992 and aims to "influence the professional development of students in health-related fields in ways that strengthen their commitment to...public service" (The Albert Schweitzer Fellowship, 2010). In recent years, it has increased the number of cities in which it operates and the number of fellows it funds. Another example is the Josiah Macy Foundation, which seeks to improve public health through supporting changes in health professional education (The Josiah Macy Foundation, 2010). Since the 1970s, the foundation has provided up to 50 grants each year to fund projects in five key areas, one of which is education for the care of the underserved. In recent years, funded projects have focused increasingly on training students in advocacy and community engagement; in 2010 they supported a third-year longitudinal clerkship experience at Mount Sinai School of Medicine that intended to "teach humanism, advocacy, and interdisciplinary medical care in the context of working longitudinally with the disenfranchised." One last example is the Institute on Medicine as a Profession Program (IMAP), which is funded with seed money from George Soros' Open Society Institute to train physicians in principles of professionalism and advocacy. Between 1999 and 2007, the IMAP Physician Advocacy Fellowship program supported 44 physicians as they developed or enhanced their advocacy skills by implementing a project in partnership with an advocacy organization. Their diverse projects addressed issues including Medicaid coverage and enrollment, health care access, pediatric oral health, and prison health care (Institute on Medicine as a Profession Program, 2011). As these large, forward-looking foundations increasingly fund such advocacy work, it becomes clear that they view health care professionals as pivotal to the process of social change.

WHAT YOU BRING TO THE TABLE, AND WILL TAKE FROM THIS BOOK

Health care has changed dramatically over the past several decades. As median survival ages have risen, health care professionals have developed new treatments for nonfatal diseases as well as fatal ones. Of course, health care has become more technical with, for example, the programming of cochlear implants and electrical stimulators that aid in stroke recovery. Despite all the wizardry of technology, however, providers still must take into account the personal, social, and financial situations of their patients. As we do so, we confront the health disparities that motivate many of us to fight social injustice and work for change.

Before you begin your journey, we suggest you make a list of the causes that led you to pick up this book. In fact, as part of one of our advocacy courses at the University of California, San Francisco, we have our trainees in child psychiatry review the personal statements they wrote at the time they applied to the program to help them reconnect with their expressed ideals. Keep these visions in mind; they will serve as a moral compass amid the turbulence of competing forces and interests. These visions, along with your perseverance, are what you bring to the table.

Now, keep reading, and you will learn to channel your passion by means of effective strategies, and to think like a seasoned advocate. You will begin to think explicitly in terms of constituents of advocacy, those whom you wish to benefit. You will come to identify the stakeholders; some may not be immediately apparent, but could be powerful and effective allies in your efforts. You will begin to view advocacy efforts systematically in terms of specific targets of your efforts and desired outcomes. Then, your passion will combine with productivity. In short, you will bring effect to your cause.

REFLECTION QUESTIONS

1. Why am I reading this book? What motivated me to learn more about advocacy?
2. What is compelling about my background that gives me enhanced credibility for the issues that interest me?
3. What specific talents, beyond my clinical training, do I bring to advocacy work?

PRACTICE MAKES PERFECT

Consider an advocacy issue that interests you:
1. Who are the main constituents? Who are all the other stakeholders?
2. What outcomes would be desirable and how will you know when you have achieved them?
3. What are the obstacles you can think of? In other words, why has this issue not moved forward already?

REFERENCES

American Dental Association. (n.d.). Retrieved May 11, 2011, from www.ada.org/fluoride.aspx
American Medical Association. (n.d.). Retrieved May 11, 2011, from www.ama-assn.org/ama/pub/physician-resources/public-health/promoting-healthy-lifestyles.page?
American Nurse's Association. (n.d.). Retrieved May 11, 2011, from www.rnaction.org/site/PageServer?pagename=nstat_take_action_healthcare_reform&ct=1l&ct=1&ct=1

Association of American Medical Colleges. (n.d.). *The road to becoming a doctor*. Retrieved May 11, 2011, from www.aamc.org

Aston-Brown, R. E. (2009). Utilizing public health clinics for service-learning rotations in dental hygiene: A four-year retrospective study. *Journal of Dental Education, 73*(3), 358–374.

Becker, H. S., & Geer, B. (1958). The fate of idealism in medical school. *American Sociological Review, 23*(1), 50–56.

Breidbart, E. (August 17, 2007). Med student struggles to preserve her idealism. *CNN.com*. Retrieved May 11, 2011, from http://edition.cnn.com/2007/HEALTH/08/16/med.student.essay/index.html

Campbell, A. (2010). The medical mission and modern cultural competency training. *Journal of American College of Surgeons, 212*(1), 124–129.

Davis, E. (2007). Serving the public good: Challenges of dental education in the twenty-first century. *Journal of Dental Education, 71*(8), 1009–1019.

Godkin, M. A., & Savageau, J. (2003). The effect of medical students' international experiences on attitudes toward serving underserved multicultural populations. *Family Medicine, 35*(4), 273–278.

Griffith, C. H., & Wilson, J. F. (2001). The loss of student idealism in the 3rd-year clinical clerkships. *Evaluation and the Health Professions, 24*, 61–71.

Griffith, C. H., & Wilson, J. F. (2003). The loss of idealism throughout internship. *Evaluation and the Health Professions, 26*, 415–426.

Hartocollis, A. (September 2, 2010). In medical school shift, meeting patients on day 1. *The New York Times*. Retrieved May 11, 2011, from www.nytimes.com/2010/09/03/nyregion/03medschool.html?src=me&ref=general

Hood, J. G. (2009). Service learning in dental education: Meeting needs and challenges. *Journal of Dental Education, 73*(4), 454–463.

Institute on Medicine as a Profession Program. (2011). Retrieved May 11, 2011, from www.imapny.org/physician_advocacy/advocacy-fellows

Keselyak, N. (2007). Evaluation of an academic service-learning course on special needs patients for dental hygiene students: A qualitative study. *Journal of Dental Education, 71*(3), 378–392.

Kidder, T. (2003). *Mountains beyond mountains*. New York, NY: Random House.

Liaison Committee on Medical Education. (2010). *Functions and structure of a medical school*. Retrieved May 11, 2011, from www.lcme.org/functions2010jun.pdf

Maben, J. (2007). The sustainability of ideals, values, and the nursing mandate: Evidence from a longitudinal qualitative study. *Nursing Inquiry, 14*(2), 99–113.

Nation, C., Gersternberger, A., & Bullard, D. (2007). Preparing for change: The plan, the promise, and the parachute. *Academic Medicine, 82*(12), 1139–1144.

National Center for Medical-Legal Partnership. Retrieved May 11, 2011, from www.medical-legalpartnership.org/

PRIME-US, University of California School of Medicine. Retrieved from http://medschool.ucsf.edu/prime/

Random House Webster's College Dictionary (2nd ed.). (1998). New York, NY: Random House.

Rezler, A. G. (1974). Attitude changes during medical school: A review of the literature. *Journal of Medical Education, 49*(11), 1023–1030.

Shaywitz, D. A., & Ausiello, D. (2002). A chance for Western physicians to give—and receive. *American Journal of Medicine, 113*(4), 354–357.

Shem, S. (1988). *House of god.* New York, NY: Dell.

Smith, J. K., & Weaver, D. B. (2006). Capturing medical student idealism. *Annals of Family Medicine, 4*(Suppl. 1), S32–S37.

Sorrel, A. L. (February 21, 2011). Doctor-lawyer advocacy: When medicine isn't enough. *American Medical News.* Retrieved May 11, 2011, from www.amaassn.org/amednews/2011/02/21/prsa0221.htm

Spickard, A., Gabbe, S., & Christensen, J. (2002). Mid-career burnout in generalist and specialist physicians. *Journal of the American Medical Association, 288*(12), 1447–1450.

The Albert Schweitzer Fellowship. (2010). Retrieved May 11, 2011, from www.schweitzerfellowship.org/features/us/

The Commonwealth Fund. (2003). Envisioning the future of academic health centers. *The final report of the Commonwealth Fund Task Force on Academic Health Centers.* Retrieved May 11, 2011, from www.commonwealthfund.org/usr_doc/ahc_envisioningfuture_600.pdf?section=4039

The Josiah Macy Foundation. (2010). *Our priorities.* Retrieved May 11, 2011, from www.josiahmacyfoundation.org/priorities

Tryssenaar, J. (1999). The lived experience of becoming an occupational therapist. *The British Journal of Occupational Therapy, 62*(3), 107–112.

Wear, D., & Kuczewki, M. G. (2008). Perspective: Medical students' perceptions of the poor: What impact can medical education have? *Academic Medicine, 83*(7), 639–645.

Wolf, T. M. (1989). A retrospective study of attitude change during medical education. *Medical Education, 23*(1), 19–23.

Vaida, B. (January 7, 2011). Doctors continued to spend big on lobbying in 2010. *Kaiser Health News.* Retrieved May 11, 2011, from www.kaiserhealthnews.org/Stories/2011/January/27/ama-lobbying.aspx

2

Learning How to Advocate: Perspectives From Medical Educators

JOHN Q. YOUNG, FUMI MITSUISHI, AND LOWELL TONG

> *The only person who is educated is the one who has learned how to learn and change.*—Carl Rogers

THE ADVOCACY IMPERATIVE

The U.S. health care system faces unprecedented challenges. A significant proportion of our population lacks financial access to health care, and even those who do possess health insurance can face significant barriers to care (Davis, Schoen, & Stremikis, 2010). While the Patient Protection and Affordable Care Act of March 2010 promises to reduce some of the barriers to care, other profound challenges persist. The cost of health care continues to skyrocket. Medical expenditures far outpace inflation and are expected to surpass 19% of Gross Domestic Product by 2019 (Sisko et al., 2010).

Despite spending about twice as much on health care as other developed countries, health outcomes in the United States are unsatisfactory by many standards (Davis et al., 2010; Ginsburg et al., 2008). A World Health Organization report in 2000 ranked the United States 37th on health care quality (World Health Organization, The World Health Report 2000-Health Systems: Improving Performance). A 2007 Commonwealth Fund Report ranked the U.S. health care system last or next-to-last on five dimensions of a high-performance health system based on quality, access, efficiency, equity, and healthy lives (Davis et al., 2010). Concerns about the safety and quality of health care continue to mount. The 1999 watershed report by the Institute of Medicine,

To err is human, estimated that nearly 100,000 preventable deaths occur in U.S. hospitals each year (Institute of Medicine, *To err is human: Building a safer health system*). Approximately 15 million incidents of medical harm occur every year in the United States, such as medication errors, wrong-site surgeries, iatrogenic infection, and missed diagnoses. A recent RAND study concluded that patients receive care that meets generally accepted standards only 55% of the time (McGlynn et al., 2003) and patients receive recommended pharmacologic care only a little more than 60% of the time (Shrank et al., 2006). These disparities in care exist across conditions (preventive, acute, and chronic), patient populations (age, ethnicity, and socioeconomic status), and geography (Asch et al., 2006; Wennbert, Fisher, Goodman, & Skinner, 2008). When specific improvements in care are developed, widespread adoption by individual clinicians can take years; some studies estimate it to take 10 to 20 years (Berwick, 2003; Institute of Medicine, 2001). Taken together, the emerging picture suggests that health care in America is unduly expensive, unreliable, and sometimes even unsafe.

As a result, health professionals and the systems in which they work will face increasing pressures to provide *higher* quality and safer health care at a *lower* cost to *more* people (Institute of Medicine, 2001). The Institute of Medicine has defined six dimensions of quality that a future health care system must possess: Safe, effective, family-centered, timely, efficient, and equal. These demands, often conflicting and sometimes irreconcilable, will place great burdens on our health professionals and their patients. To accomplish these goals will require a fundamental redesign of how health care is delivered (Bohmer, 2010).

These redesigns offer an amazing opportunity to imagine and create a health care system that is far more humane and effective. Health professionals are key front-line stakeholders—and a crucial resource—in this process. We possess on-the-ground knowledge of patient experiences and the science of care. We know firsthand the current gaps in care and the impact on patients and providers. We have the lived-experience of operating within our complex system of care, which means that we have intimate knowledge of its constraints and opportunities to promote a supportive and sustainable work environment. Unless health professionals learn how to advocate effectively, dramatic changes will proceed *without* our input, values, and experience—this may not only make our professional experiences less rewarding, but degrade the clinician–patient relationship and the quality of care. It is therefore critical that health professionals possess the skills and capabilities to lead and shape this change process. When advocacy reignites our idealism, we may even discover renewed meaning and purpose in our professional lives.

THE ADVOCACY SKILLS GAP

To meet this and other important challenges ripe for advocacy, we must address a fundamental gap in the skills that health care professionals typically possess. As it stands, medical education across the continuum, from undergraduate medical education (UME) through graduate medical education (GME) to continuing medical education (CME) provides minimal, often cursory, training in advocacy. Other health professions, such as nursing, do better, but even there advocacy is a relatively underrepresented topic and skill. For example, while "advocacy" is considered to be a core competency in nursing, it specifically refers to patient advocacy (e.g., speaking out for patients, act on unmet needs of patients) (Hanks, 2010) and thus does not encompass other forms of advocacy, such as influencing state policy (Mallik, 1997; Spenceley, Reutter, & Allen, 2006). In addition, the instruction on patient advocacy tends to be "haphazard" and not methodically taught (Foley, Minick, & Kee, 2002).

One fundamental problem is rooted in the fact that we, as health professionals, are generally trained to work with the individual rather than with groups or systems, the discipline of social work being an important exception. In 1999, the Accreditation Council for Graduate Medical Education (ACGME), the regulatory body for graduate medical education in the United States, adopted systems-based practice (SBP) as one of the six competency domains for physicians. This mandate elevated the importance of working within systems to improve care and has led to some increased attention to advocacy and related skills. In fact, all pediatrics residencies must now provide basic training in advocacy. However, progress has been slow and incorporation of systems-based practice into traditional clinical curricula has been a challenging proposition.

As a result, SBP is the least likely competency to be formally incorporated into a medical curriculum (Colbert, Ogden, Ownby, & Bowe, 2011; Ziegelstein & Fiebach, 2004). This may not be surprising given that curricula in the health professions focus on knowledge of biomedical science and clinical skills related to the care of individual patients. Rarely do these curricula focus on the science of quality, health administration and policy, or organizational change processes. Physicians and physicians-in-training are evaluated and advanced on the basis of the individual, not cohorts or teams. It is important to note that SBP, which is defined by the ACGME as the ability to respond "to the larger context and system of health care," and "to call effectively on other resources in the system to provide optimal health care," (ACGME, n.d.) is necessary but not sufficient for effective advocacy. In addition, though one of the ways in which resident physicians demonstrate SBP is by advocating for "quality patient care and optimal patient care systems," how a training program can develop this skill in its residents and determine when the skill that has been learned has not been delineated.

Advocacy often requires a health professional to "cross borders" and travel into unfamiliar territory. Indeed, in order to be effective advocates, clinicians need to learn about power, organizational change, and politics, to understand how to influence processes that allocate important resources. In addition, there may also be an "attitude gap." For example, medical training typically encourages a culture of compliance and self-sacrifice and discourages argumentative stances or vocal complaining. This attitude may be supported by the tradition of training centered on an apprenticeship model, where one learns by imitation rather than encouragement to innovate. Lastly, though some health professionals understand patient advocacy and even systems improvement to be a part of their mission, this view is not shared by all health professionals. Often, the recognition that advocacy is a formal "task" for a health professional is lacking. And even when this awareness exists, health professionals often report feeling intimidated or lacking in confidence about the activities surrounding advocacy (Roth et al., 2004).

WHAT NEEDS TO BE LEARNED?

If health professionals are to meet the challenges of redesigning health care, we will need to become effective advocates. Yet, few of us have been prepared for this role. Thus, a critical task centers on how we develop and participate in programs that effectively train us for advocacy. These programs must deliver the right content. In a study on child advocacy training curricula for pediatrics residency programs, the authors surveyed a number of national experts to agree on a working definition of advocacy and arrived at this working definition: "To speak up, to plead, or to champion for a cause while applying professional expertise and leadership to support efforts on individual (patient or family), community, and legislative/policy levels, which result in the improved quality of life for individuals, families, or communities" (Wright, Katcher, et al., 2005; Wright, Moreno, et al., 2005). The first part of the definition emphasizes the active process of speaking up, which makes sense given that the etymology of "advocate" can be traced back to the Latin roots of *"ad"* and *"vocare,"* which means "to call" or "to invoke." The term was initially applied to a person called upon to plead another's case.

The chapters that follow cover the many different advocacy strategies and tactics. The ways in which one goes about championing or pleading a case are extremely varied (Altman, Balcazar, Fawcett, Seekins, & Young, 1994). The broad spectrum of advocacy activities include documenting the problem, framing the issue effectively, identifying

TABLE 2.1
Examples of Topics for an Advocacy Curriculum

Define the problem	Needs assessment: Collecting and analyzing data to understand the nature, scope, and magnitude of the problem.
	Identify the causes of the problem and its key contributing factors. Methods to aid this process are many, such as: A root cause analysis, which iteratively asks "why or what caused…," and the fishbone or Ishikawa diagram, which breaks down the problem into its component of "man, methods, machines, materials, measurements and environments."
Choose the aim	Select an objective that is achievable, measurable, and relevant (i.e., actually addresses the problem).
Develop and implement the strategy	Identify the target audience(s): Understanding where "the power" lies and identifying entities or individuals with decision-making power or potential influence over those with power.
	Develop and deliver advocacy messages: Shaping a message that speaks to the audience(s), including selecting appropriate data to support an argument, making persuasive arguments, choosing metaphors and examples strategically, and learning to strategically use the media.
	Build coalitions and fundraise: Networking, team and alliance building, and financial management.
Assess the progress	Evaluate the advocacy effort, then return to step 1 and modify as appropriate until the aim has been achieved!

Source: Adapted from Altman et al. (1994).

underlying causes and those with the power and/or authority to change the situation, verbal persuasion, nonviolent protest, boycotts, applying economic pressure, using the media, filing a formal complaint, initiating legal action, writing letters to decision-makers, testifying, participating in lobbying activities, piloting an alternative approach, celebrating a positive change, and so on. As noted in Chapter 1, we start and restart our journey as advocates by returning to the place where we identify our personal passions that will motivate us through successes and setbacks. Next, regardless of the causes and strategies our passions lead us to pursue, we must develop core skills, including those delineated in Table 2.1.

EDUCATIONAL STRATEGIES THAT DO NOT WORK

As discussed above, our effort to learn advocacy depends upon our ability to learn the right content—in this case, the right knowledge, skills, and attitudes. To learn the right content, we must choose to participate in educational activities that work; that is, help us learn how *to be advocates,* and then to actually "walk the talk," or put those skills into practice in order to improve outcomes. It turns out this is no simple task.

Continuing medical education (CME), as part of the life-long learning spectrum, represents a primary strategy for the ongoing education of independent practitioners. The AMA defines CME as "educational activities that serve to maintain, develop, or increase the knowledge, skills, and professional performance and relationships a physician uses to provide services for patients, the public, or the profession." Unfortunately, the prevailing approaches to continuing (and, for that matter, most) education in the health professions are based on teaching methods that are ineffective. This framework relies on process requirements (e.g., number of hours of CME per year) and content (e.g., pain management) (Davis et al., 1999). The instructional methods are typically based on lectures, often with audio-visual presentations (e.g., PowerPoint presentations), and printed materials (e.g., guidelines or handouts of a PowerPoint presentation). Such CME activities lead to some knowledge gains, though these gains tend to be poorly sustained (Bordage, Carlin, & Mazmanian, 2009). More significantly, these strategies have limited impact on physician behavior change or patient outcomes (Davis & Taylor-Vaisey, 1997). Davis et al. found in their review of randomized controlled trials of formal CME activities (didactic, interactive, and mixed methods) that studies comparing didactics to no intervention showed no improvement in physician performance (Davis et al., 1999). One of these studies randomly assigned 174 physicians to one of three intervention groups: A standard three-hour seminar on the national guidelines for high cholesterol monitoring and management, an intensive intervention composed of the standard intervention with follow-up seminars and free office material, or a control group. A chart review of patients of the physicians who participated was conducted a year and a half after the intervention, and it was found that there was no difference in screening rate or compliance with the guidelines between either intervention groups and the control (Browner, Baron, Solkowitz, Adler, & Gullion, 1994). In the same vein, a review of systematic reviews looking at the effectiveness of multiple CME educational tools and techniques found that didactic presentations and distribution of printed material have little or no beneficial effect in changing physician practice and patient outcomes (Bloom, 2005).

Given the limited efficacy of traditional continuing education approaches, it is no surprise that innovations, even when backed with evidence, take a decade or more to be adopted, and that the gap between best practice and actual practice grows over the course of one's career. Importantly, if we are to train health professionals to be effective advocates, we must use more effective pedagogies—pedagogies informed by the learning sciences.

EDUCATIONAL STRATEGIES THAT WORK

The learning sciences have identified the educational principles associated with curricula that work, that is, effectively engaging health professionals in learning new knowledge, skills, and attitudes and, ultimately, changing what we do (Green & Ellis, 1997; Mann, 2002; Mazmanian & Davis, 2002). Table 2.2 highlights selected principles to consider as you develop your own strategy for learning advocacy, create advocacy curricula for others, or even craft messages for the targets of our advocacy work for those who, after all, are also learners! Keep these principles in mind as you move through the chapters that follow. In fact, most of the "Practice Makes Perfect" learning activities that appear at the end of each chapter are based upon these principles.

Consistent with these educational principles, systematic reviews of continuing education interventions have identified a number of common themes (Mansouri & Lockyer, 2007; Marinopoulos et al., 2007). Print media is less effective than trainings delivered in person, and multimedia generally seems to be more effective than single media. In addition, interactive techniques (e.g., simulation, role play, small group project) are more effective than noninteractive ones (e.g., lectures), and multiple exposures more so than single exposures. Table 2.3 summarizes the different CME components that may also be included in an educational activity related to advocacy. No two learners are the same. Which of these features are most consistently effective for your individual learning style?

Flexible, web-based CME represents a relatively new medium with widespread and increasing use. From 1998 to 2003, the number of internet-based CMEs increased 700%, compared to a 40% increase in non-internet-based CME. Also, by 2003, 45% to 64% of MDs participated in internet-based CMEs. There is a growing body of evidence about the effectiveness of web-based CME (Casebeer et al., 2003; Crenshaw et al., 2010; Fordis et al., 2005). Web-based health professional education offers greater flexibility with timing of training, improved availability to learners who are geographically dispersed, reduced travel expenses and time, and therefore overall more accessibility for the busy professional. It also provides greater adaptability to the learner's personal style by allowing flexibility in sequencing, thus more closely adhering to learning principles. Its potential for interactivity can be used to connect the content to the context where it is applied and for dialogue (real time or asynchronous) between learners, or learners and instructors. Lastly, it has the capability for multimedia and multifaceted instruction. In a randomized controlled trial that compared web-based CME to in-person CME, subjects assigned to the online module, though less comfortable with the technology than those assigned to the live module, demonstrated more significant change in practice behavior (Fordis et al., 2005).

TABLE 2.2
Selected Principles to Guide Learning How to Advocate

Activate prior knowledge	Each health professional brings prior knowledge and experiences, which form the basis for new learning. Effective training connects new learning to prior knowledge. Exercises that activate prior knowledge include: Discussion, review, questioning, and reflective exercises.
Elaborate new knowledge	Process of actively working with (e.g., note taking and study), discussing (e.g., small groups), and practicing new knowledge, skills, and attitudes, especially in new situations (e.g., everyday practice or role play).
Learning in context	Learning that occurs in relevant situation facilitates "encoding" that is readily retrieved and applied—the learning situation should approximate as much as possible the actual situations in which it will be applied (e.g., testifying, talking with the press, writing a position paper).
Knowledge/ skill transfer	Learning is context specific. We often do not transfer what is learned in the educational setting (e.g., classroom, workshop, conference) to new situations in our everyday practice. As learners, we must work with many different examples to help facilitate transfer.
Observation	This reflects the basic principle that underlies the importance of role modeling and its powerful effects on how we, as learners, think, act, and develop. In addition to direct observation, hearing the advocacy stories of others can help inspire and facilitate elaboration and transfer.
Feedback	Learning is facilitated by feedback from peers or instructors that is specific, based on direct observation, in close proximity to the event, both reenforcing and corrective, situated in a safe interpersonal setting, incorporates self-reflection/assessment, and ends with a specific plan for further growth.
Self-efficacy	Self-efficacy is our perception of our ability to perform a given activity and is informed by experience, observation of others' abilities, our own feelings, and encouragement from others. Self-efficacy influences the kinds and difficulty of goals that a learner sets and our persistence in achieving those goals. This highlights the importance of clear expectations, feedback, and encouragement.
Learning in the workplace	Learning occurs through interaction with people in the workplace through "talking about" and "listening to talk" about the framing and solution of practice problems. This highlights the importance of gradated learning, in which the participant moves from more peripheral participation to more central involvement.
Self-direction	This process starts with self-assessment of your knowledge gap, followed by learner-owned curricula and goal setting, and ends with evaluation of learning through self-reflection about learning objective attainment.

Source: Adapted from Mann (2002).

TABLE 2.3
Features of Continuing Education Programs

Media Method	Instructional Method	Simulation Types	Timing
In-person	Lecture	Full simulation	One time
Computer based, offline	Audience response system	Partial simulation	Repetitive
	Case-based learning		Sequencing
Internet, real time (streaming)	Apprenticeship	Computer simulation	Fixed vs. flexible
	Demonstration	Virtual reality	
Internet, not real time	Discussion group	Role play	
	Feedback		
Video	Lecture		
Audio	Mentor/coach		
Handheld	Readings		
Print	Reflection		
	Role play		
	Simulation		
	Writing		

PUTTING LEARNING PRINCIPLES INTO PRACTICE

The educational principles and techniques highlighted in Tables 2.2 and 2.3 have a number of practical implications for how to design or participate in effective advocacy training programs. How to apply these principles becomes clearer when viewed through the broader framework of "structure, content, process, and outcomes" (Table 2.4). When designing curriculum, defining "outcomes" should be the first step. Training programs should first have clear and measurable goals: Learning objectives relevant to and shaped by the intended learners. Once this step is achieved, the content of what needs to be taught can be identified, and the process (instructional method) most congruent with achieving the learning objective can be chosen (Kern, Thomas, & Hughes, 2009). It will be helpful to characterize the learning goal as "cognitive" (knowledge), "affective" (attitude), or "psychomotor" (skills or behavior) in order to arrive at the best-matched educational method. To illustrate, if the learning objective is effective team or coalition building to organize an advocacy effort, there may be knowledge (cognitive) goals about the principles of group dynamics that could be achieved through readings and lectures. In addition, the affective objective of engendering a collaborative attitude may be facilitated by a practice exercise where each member of the team assumes semi-scripted roles within the group, afterwards reflects on the

TABLE 2.4
Proposed Features of Advocacy Training Programs for Health Professionals

Structure	Identify target audience
	Components: Awareness, understanding, practical skills, and experience (Rudolf, 2003)
	Outcome based instead of time based
Content	Three levels: Patient/individual/bedside; community; and policy/legislature (Wright, Moreno et al., 2005)
	Generated by a need and from the learner's own experience
	Focused on specific, measurable competencies
Process	Interactive, simulation based, repeated exposures, longitudinal contact, experiential and project based, community networking and partnership, project monitoring and self-reflection process, instructors with a variety of expertise and background
Outcomes	Actual skills or behavior. System changes, patient outcomes. Sustainability of the project or endurance of changes

experience, and shares internal reactions during a facilitated discussion session. Lastly, there may be psychomotor objectives, such as changing a team member's behavior, that impedes the team building process. For example, one member may have the tendency to be passively disengaged and another the tendency to overtake the group's discussion. To address this issue, a group-based feedback process embedded in serial real-life experiences of working as a team would be helpful.

Once the learning outcome has been defined, we can consider how best to structure learning experience. There are many important aspects to the structure of a curriculum, but just as in an advocacy campaign, the intended audience is crucial. A curriculum designed to address the needs of a mixed versus a homogeneous group of health professionals, or of individuals broadly interested in advocacy work versus those with a clear advocacy objective in mind, will need to differ significantly. In general, the structure should be comprised of four broad components: (a) *awareness* (self reflection, background information search on topic), (b) *understanding* (developing a system to identify underlying causes, didactics on political process, direct contact with successful advocates), (c) *practical skills* (learning how to do stakeholder analysis or how to interface with the media—TV, radio, press releases, letters), and (d) *experience* (developing a plan for action and taking the next step) (Rudolf, 2003). Because the ultimate product of an advocacy curriculum is effective advocacy work, the structure of the curriculum should be experiential and shaped around results, such as a project or an observable product rather than focused primarily on the acquisition of knowledge. Establishing the feasibility of an educational strategy based on the resources available will define what can be implemented and therefore its structure. Resources to consider are faculty and learner time, motivation, level of experience, finances, materials, and space.

For any given advocacy goal, an effective curriculum must convey the relevant knowledge—such knowledge it is the grounding basis upon which budding advocates will build their understanding of the problem, its solution, and the strategy to bridge the two. There are three levels of knowledge to consider when designing advocacy trainings: the level of the individual (e.g., patient), the level of the community, and the even more encompassing level of public policy (e.g., state legislature) (Wright, Moreno et al., 2005)

In terms of process, when possible, curricula should link the newly learned skills to prior knowledge or skills that the health professionals possess. For example, the importance and capacity of using the types of language that will engage the general public when communicating with the press can be compared to the importance of modifying how we explain treatment options when educating a patient. When the educational objective is especially complex and encompasses several domains, as is the case for advocacy training, educational strategies should utilize multiple mediums (e.g., video, in-person, and written) and interactive, highly engaging methods. As described in Table 2.3, multiple instructional methods can be used to this end, and the example of audience response system provides a perfect illustration. An audience response system is an innovative teaching technology that can be used in combination with lectures or discussion groups. This computerized feedback tool allows a large group of learners to answer an instructor's question en masse. The responses are collated and presented on a screen and at times used by the instructor to alter the teaching content based on audience response, thus engaging the learner's existing knowledge, shaping the learning process according to learners' preferences, interests, skills/knowledge levels, and adding interactivity to effectively engage learners.

You can learn advocacy skills optimally through learning activities that simulate as closely as possible the actual advocacy task or skill and incorporate feedback. In role-play, a type of simulation, learners act out an assigned position or role in front of other learners. Frequently, a discussion follows, where learners are asked to reflect on their experience or to provide feedback on ways to improve the interaction. For example, training on media advocacy might have learners in small groups craft a press release, followed by each learner conducting a simulated 5-minute press conference while other group members play the role of the press. The session could be tape recorded and then reviewed in the small group which then gives the learner direct feedback. Role plays, as illustrated in this example, are helpful in meeting affective and psychomotor learning objectives because they provide the opportunity to simulate an interaction, the space to reflect on the reactions provoked, and the chance to receive or provide feedback to impart a change in attitude and behavior. These can be powerful learning experiences and motivators for future learning.

Effective training programs will occur over time with repeated exposures within a relatively stable community of learners/practitioners that provide ongoing support and accountability. They will be linked to actual products realized in terms of clinician skills or behavior, systemic changes, and measurable patient or population health outcomes (e.g., less medical errors, increased availability of culturally and linguistically appropriate care, increased funding for preventative health screens). It is also important to keep in mind the sustainability of the project or the endurance of the changes. As in any change process, monitoring each of these is of utmost importance, as it will provide a feedback loop to encourage further growth on the path to build a community of advocates.

CASE STUDY: THE INSTITUTE FOR HEALTHCARE IMPROVEMENT

The Institute for Healthcare Improvement (IHI) is a nonprofit organization based in Boston that has had a significant impact on health care quality and safety, both here in the United States and around the world (Institute for Healthcare Improvement, 2011). IHI has launched multiple voluntary initiatives that have changed how hospitals and clinics deliver care and, in so doing, saved millions of lives. A key element of IHI's success lies in how it has trained health care professionals to become effective advocates and leaders of change. A review of its website (www.ihi.org) illustrates many of the learning strategies described above. For example, IHI's Knowledge Center provides access to the 'right content' via resources such as practical tools, change ideas, measures to guide improvement, white papers, and improvement stories. This content is conveyed in multiple formats, including print, audio, and visuals. In addition, IHI offers online courses that can be taken at any time and in-person seminars and conferences. To support the translation of the newly acquired skills into action, IHI facilitates a number of collaboratives and networks that create a learning community for a defined period of time. Entry requires a commitment to participate, meet predefined expectations, sometimes pay tuition, and carry out a project in one's own home institution. These communities link people across organizations that then provide each other with ongoing support and accountability and repeated exposure to key content and skills over time. These communities are organized around real-life projects with specific goals and aims. Finally, IHI leads strategic initiatives that test the next wave of innovations to be deployed throughout health care. While these initiatives are not open for enrollment, IHI invites all to learn from these efforts and models by sharing their successes and failures. As we choose how best to learn new skills or train others, IHI is a good example of an organization that is training health professionals using strategies that work.

CONCLUSION

Endeavoring to meet the needs of our patients and the challenges of our health care system, we as health professionals must learn effective ways to advocate for meaningful change. This will require us to acquire new skills and to train others in these skills. As we do so, our success will in part depend on choosing effective learning structures and processes to learn the right content in order to achieve the outcomes we are most passionate about.

REFLECTION QUESTIONS

1. What "causes" or "issues" are you most passionate about?
2. Who else is likely to share this passion?
3. What type of advocacy activities are of most interest to you? What advocacy skill would you like to further hone?
4. What is the next step you can take to enhance your skill in this activity?

PRACTICE MAKES PERFECT

1. Engage and persuade a decision maker: Practice the "elevator talk" by delivering your argument out loud for a given cause in under 2 minutes.
2. Create a media pitch: Develop three metaphors, analogies or "interesting facts" that you can use to dramatize the importance of a given cause. For example, the Institute of Medicine illustrated the magnitude of a 100,000 preventable deaths a year by equating this to a jumbo jet crash every day for a year.

REFERENCES

ACGME. (n.d.). Retrieved from www.acgme.org/acWebsite/navPages/common pr_documents/IVA5f_EducationalProgram_ACGMECompetencies_SBP_Explanation.pdf

Altman, D. G., Balcazar, F. E., Fawcett, S. B., Seekins, T., & Young, J. Q. (1994). *Public Health Advocacy: Creating community change to improve health.* Palo Alto, CA: Leland Stanford Junior University.

Asch, S. M., Kerr, E. A., Keesey, J., Adams, J. L., Setodji, C. M., Malik, S., & McGlynn E. A. (2006). Who is at greatest risk for receiving poor-quality health care? *The New England Journal of Medicine, 354*(11), 1147–1156.

Berwick, D. M. (2003). Disseminating innovations in health care. *Journal of the American Medical Association, 289*(15), 1969–1975.

Bloom, B. S. (2005). Effects of continuing medical education on improving physician clinical care and patient health: A review of systematic reviews. *International Journal of Technology Assessment in Health Care, 21*(3), 380–385.

Bohmer, R. M. (2010). Fixing health care on the front lines. *Harvard Business Review, 88*(4), 62–69.

Bordage, G., Carlin, B., & Mazmanian, P. E. (2009). Continuing medical education effect on physician knowledge: Effectiveness of continuing medical education: American College of Chest Physicians Evidence-Based Educational Guidelines. *Chest, 135*(3 Suppl.), 29S–36S.

Browner, W. S., Baron, R. B., Solkowitz, S., Adler, L. J., & Gullion, D. S. (1994). Physician management of hypercholesterolemia. A randomized trial of continuing medical education. *The Western Journal of Medicine, 161*(6), 572–578.

Casebeer, L. L., Strasser, S. M., Spettell, C. M., Wall, T. C., Weissman, N., Ray, M. N., & Allison, J. J. (2003). Designing tailored Web-based instruction to improve practicing physicians' preventive practices. *Journal of Medical Internet Research, 5*(3), e20.

Colbert, C. Y., Ogden, P. E., Ownby, A. R., & Bowe, C. (2011). Systems-based practice in graduate medical education: Systems thinking as the missing foundational construct. *Teaching and Learning in Medicine, 23*(2), 179–185.

Crenshaw, K., Curry, W., Salanitro, A. H., Safford, M. M., Houston, T. K., Allison, J. J., & Estrada, C. A. (2010). Is physician engagement with Web-based CME associated with patients' baseline hemoglobin A1c levels? The Rural Diabetes Online Care study. *Academic Medicine, 85*(9), 1511–1517.

Davis, D., O'Brien, M. A., Freemantle, N., Wolf, F. M., Mazmanian, P., & Taylor-Vaisey, A. (1999). Impact of formal continuing medical education: Do conferences, workshops, rounds, and other traditional continuing education activities change physician behavior or health care outcomes? *Journal of the American Medical Association, 282*(9), 867–874.

Davis, D. A., & Taylor-Vaisey, A. (1997). Translating guidelines into practice. A systematic review of theoretic concepts, practical experience and research evidence in the adoption of clinical practice guidelines. *Canadian Medical Association Journal, 157*(4), 408–416.

Davis, K., Schoen, C., & Stremikis, K. (2010). *Mirror Mirror on the Wall: How the Performance of the US Health Care System Compares Internationally.* New York, NY: The Commonwealth Fund.

Foley, B. J., Minick, M. P., & Kee, C. C. (2002). How nurses learn advocacy. *Journal of Nursing Scholarship, 34*(2), 181–186.

Fordis, M., King, J. E., Ballantyne, C. M., Jones, P. H., Schneider, K. H., Spann, S. J.,...Greisinger, A. J. (2005). Comparison of the instructional efficacy of Internet-based CME with live interactive CME workshops: A randomized controlled trial. *Journal of the American Medical Association, 294*(9), 1043–1051.

Ginsburg, J. A., Doherty, R. B., Ralston, J. F., Jr., Senkeeto, N., Cooke, M., Cutler, C.,...Stubbs, J. W. (2008). Achieving a high-performance health care system with universal access: What the United States can learn from other countries. *Annals of Internal Medicine, 148*(1), 55–75.

Green, M. L., & Ellis, P. J. (1997). Impact of an evidence-based medicine curriculum based on adult learning theory. *Journal of General Internal Medicine, 12*(12), 742–750.

Hanks, R. G. (2010). Development and testing of an instrument to measure protective nursing advocacy. *Nursing Ethics, 17*(2), 255–267.

Institute for Healthcare Improvement (2011). Retrieved August 31, 2011, from www.ihi.org

Institute of Medicine. (2000). *To err is human: Building a safer health system.* Washington, DC: National Academy Press.

Institute of Medicine. (2001). *Crossing the quality chasm: A new health system for the 21st century.* Washington, DC: National Academy Press.

Kern, D. E., Thomas, P. A., & Hughes, M. T. (2009). *Curriculum development for medical education: A six-step approach* (2nd ed.). Baltimore, MD: Johns Hopkins University Press.

Mallik, M. (1997). Advocacy in nursing—A review of the literature. *Journal of Advanced Nursing, 25*(1), 130–138.

Mann, K. V. (2002). Thinking about learning: Implications for principle-based professional education. *The Journal of Continuing Education in the Health Professions, 22*(2), 69–76.

Mansouri, M., & Lockyer, J. (2007). A meta-analysis of continuing medical education effectiveness. *The Journal of Continuing Education in the Health Professions, 27*(1), 6–15.

Marinopoulos, S. S., Dorman, T., Ratanawongsa, N., Wilson, L. M., Ashar, B. H., Magaziner, J. L.,...Bass, E. B. (2007). *Effectiveness of Continuing Medical Education* (No. Publication No 07-E006). Rockville, MD: Agency for Healthcare Research and Quality.

Mazmanian, P. E., & Davis, D. A. (2002). Continuing medical education and the physician as a learner: Guide to the evidence. *Journal of the American Medical Association, 288*(9), 1057–1060.

McGlynn, E. A., Asch, S. M., Adams, J., Keesey, J., Hicks, J., DeCristofaro, A., & Kerr, E. A. (2003). The quality of health care delivered to adults in the United States. *The New England Journal of Medicine, 348*(26), 2635–2645.

Roth, E. J., Barreto, P., Sherritt, L., Palfrey, J. S., Risko, W., & Knight, J. R. (2004). A new, experiential curriculum in child advocacy for pediatric residents. *Ambulatory Pediatrics, 4*(5), 418–423.

Rudolf, M. (2003). Advocacy training for pediatricians: The experience of running a course in leeds, United Kingdom. *Pediatrics, 112*(3 Part 2), 749–751.

Shrank, W. H., Asch, S. M., Adams, J., Setodji, C., Kerr, E. A., Keesey, J., ... McGlynn, E. A. (2006). The quality of pharmacologic care for adults in the United States. *Medical Care, 44*(10), 936–945.

Sisko, A. M., Truffer, C. J., Keehan, S. P., Poisal, J. A., Clemens, M. K., & Madison, A. J. (2010). National Health Spending Projections: The Estimated Impact Of Reform Through 2019. *Health Affairs, 29*(10), 1933–1941.

Spenceley, S. M., Reutter, L., & Allen, M. N. (2006). The road less traveled: Nursing advocacy at the policy level. *Policy, Politics & Nursing Practice, 7*(3), 180–194.

Wennbert, J. E., Fisher, E. S., Goodman, D. C., & Skinner, J. S. (2008). *Ranking the care of patients with severe chronic illness. The Dartmouth atlas of health care 2008.* Dartmouth, NH: The Dartmouth Institute for Health Policy and Clinical Practice.

World Health Organization. (2000). *The world health report 2000—Health systems: Improving performance.* Retrieved from www.who.int/whr/2000/en/

Wright, C. J., Katcher, M. L., Blatt, S. D., Keller, D. M., Mundt, M. P., Botash, A. S., & Gjerde, C. L. (2005). Toward the development of advocacy training curricula for pediatric residents: A national delphi study. *Ambulatory Pediatrics, 5*(3), 165–171.

Wright, C. J., Moreno, M. A., Katcher, M. L., McIntosh, G. C., Mundt, M. P., & Corden, T. E. (2005). Development of an advocacy curriculum in a pediatric residency program. *Teaching and Learning in Medicine, 17*(2), 142–148.

Ziegelstein, R. C. & Fiebach, N. H. (2004). "The mirror" and "the village": A new method for teaching practice-based learning and improvement and systems-based practice. *Academic Medicine, 79*(1), 83–88.

3

Overview of the Political Advocacy Process

RICHARD L. BARNES

The secret of success lies in the constancy of purpose.—
Benjamin Disraeli (British author and politician, 1804–1881)

Public policy advocacy is an important tool for health professionals to affect policies that impact patient care and public health, but many do not get involved in it because they do not know what it is or how they, as individuals, can fit into the process—to make a difference. This chapter demystifies the public policy advocacy process by introducing a practical, systematic approach to policy advocacy. The focus will be on advocacy at the state and local levels, as policy advocacy at the federal level in the United States is largely carried out in private meetings between armies of lobbyists with large checks for campaign contributions and legislative staff. Also, in the last three decades, the federal government has devolved most innovative policymaking to the state and local governments; frankly, that is where all the action is. (That said, advocacy at the federal level is achievable and described in Chapter 4.) The case study in Chapter 11 demonstrates how the systematic approach to policy advocacy works in the real world.

WHAT IS POLICY ADVOCACY?

Public policy is changed in four principal ways: Legislation, administrative rulemaking, executive orders, and litigation. Executive orders have applicability only to executive branch departments and activities, but at the federal level they have been used as a catalyst for subsequent social change (i.e., President Truman desegregated the armed forces by executive order in the 1948). Litigation is a powerful advocacy tool (Anderson, 1992) and is fully discussed in Chapter 7. The 1954 U.S. Supreme Court decision ending racial segregation in public schools pushed the legislative agenda that led to the first federal civil rights act in 1963. This chapter will focus on legislation and administrative rulemaking as policymaking venues.

Political advocacy can be defined as the art of persuading policymakers to change public policy in the face of political opposition to a change. The role of the political advocate is to overcome this opposition, which comes both from policymakers and from those interests that want to maintain the status quo. To be successful in overcoming that opposition, political advocates should follow a systematic approach:

1. Conduct an objective evaluation of the challenges to the public health goal
2. Assemble an effective and committed alliance of supporting organizations
3. Design an evidence-based policy instrument to effectuate the goal
4. Develop a creative and flexible strategic plan and the means to execute it
5. Execute the strategic plan
6. Carry out an ongoing evaluation of the new policy effectiveness

These six components, taken together, are a formula for success and are discussed in detail below. Leave one component out, and the chance of success drops. While it is largely a sequential process, it is not necessarily linear; with the exception of component six, all activities, in whole or in part, may be going on simultaneously.

When activists see a problem, they want to fix it at once and often race off to the legislature for the fix without laying a proper predicate for success; often the result is failure and frustration. Instead, the policy advocate has to be persistent and patient; executing a successful policy advocacy campaign takes time given that the opposition of policymakers and defenders of the status quo must be overcome. For example, universal health care has been on the American health policy agenda for over 100 years (Quadango, 2005); the 2010 federal health care reform legislation was the first step in achieving this, but it does not provide health insurance coverage for all persons. In the end, politics determines public policy (Oliver, 2006) and politicians have struggled over whether health care should be treated as a market good or a public good (Lee, Oliver, Benjamin, & Lee, 2006). Political advocacy is what will drive the outcome of that struggle.

EVALUATING THE CHALLENGES TO THE PUBLIC HEALTH GOAL

Defining the Problem

The first step in the advocacy process is defining the problem. It is not as simple as it seems. University of California, Berkeley Professor Eugene Bardach admonishes: "Your first problem definition is a crucial step: it gives you both a reason for doing all the work necessary to complete the project and a sense of direction for your evidence-gathering activity" (Bardach, 2012, p. 1). Bardach further recommends that the problem should be defined in a way that does not include a solution; choosing a solution comes later in the policy design phase. It also helps to think of the problem in terms of an excess or deficit: "There are too many …" or "there are too few…." It may be useful to describe outcomes caused by the problem that you want to affect: "Illegal drug use increases crime." As you progress through the advocacy process, you may find that you need to amend, refine, or even completely change your problem definition. For use in this chapter, the model problem definition is: "There are too many persons in the U.S. without health insurance."

What Is Causing the Problem?

Next, an analysis of what causes the problem is needed (Stone, 1989, 2002). "Without good causal theory, it is unlikely that a policy design will be able to deliver the desired outcomes. Rather, performance measurement will remain focused on effort, because implementers and researchers will find the connection between effort and outcome so difficult to make" (Birkland, 2011, p. 241). It is also important that outcomes of the policy intervention be the focus of evaluation after implementation of the policy (Affholter, 1994).

What Is the Current Policy Environment Affecting the Problem?

To determine where you need to go to affect the problem, you must know where you are; you need a legal analysis of the current policy environment. It is advisable to consult lawyers who are experts on the problem. There are basic questions that need to be answered. Are there no existing policies that deal with the problem? Be careful here, as most problems are covered, at least in part, by some existing policies, and it is usually much easier to amend existing policy than it is to start from scratch. If there are applicable existing policies that address the problem, why do those policies fail to alleviate or eliminate the problem you have defined, or keep it from getting worse? Did those existing policies not adequately address the problem at the time they were adopted? This is a common result of the compromise that so often occurs in politics. Were those policies not implemented in the manner needed to effectively address the problem? Incomplete or ineffective implementation of policy occurs all too often. Have circumstances changed since the existing policy was adopted that results in a new problem not contemplated by the original policy? Have new methods of dealing with the problem been developed that render the existing policy obsolete? The answers to these questions will lead to more defining questions, as well as guide you in determining whether you need new legislation, amendments to existing law, revisions of existing administrative regulations, or something else.

Assessing Voter Awareness of the Problem

Vital information at this early point in an advocacy campaign is the level of voter awareness of and concern about the problem; this information is gathered through voter polling by professional pollsters. If the level of either awareness or concern is low, you should consider an educational campaign to change that. A high level of public support for dealing with the problem is important in getting policymakers to put it on their agenda for action (Mebane & Blendon, 2001). At the same time that you are educating voters, you are also educating policymakers. This triangulation of educational campaigns (by means of the media), policymakers, and voters is depicted graphically in Chapter 5.

AN ALLIANCE OF SUPPORTING ORGANIZATIONS

Building an Advocacy Alliance

Any endeavor in health policy change will likely run into powerful, well-funded opposition from entrenched interests whose history of campaign contributions to policymakers and use of well-connected lobbyists gives them influence over the policymaking process. How do you gain the political clout you will need to overcome that influence?

Political clout comes from many sources: Money, powerful connections, public credibility, name recognition, a large number of voters represented in membership, and so forth. Most advocacy campaigns require more than one organization, group, or individual to have effective political clout, so an alliance of like-minded organizations, groups, and individuals is needed. To build the alliance, first look for organizations whose agenda includes the problem you are dealing with. Identify organizations representing those who will benefit from the policy change. Your objective should be to assemble a group of organizations, groups, and individuals, each of whom has a strong interest in the goal you are seeking to achieve (Barnes, 2002; Bozlak & Kelley, 2009; deLeon & Varda, 2009; Gruen, Campbell, & Blumenthal, 2006; Sherraden, Slosar, & Sherraden, 2002). Sometimes opponents come together when there is mutual interest in the goal. The Oil Pollution Act of 1990 that mandated twin-hulled oil cargo ships in U.S. waters was the result of the combined efforts of the Alaska fishing industry and environmental groups following the *Exxon Valdez* oil spill in 1989. Prior to that, the two groups had bitter battles over the environmental impacts of fishing. Also, be mindful that some organizations have political baggage that may negatively affect your efforts; regardless of how powerful or moneyed they may be, it is usually best to leave them out of the alliance (Hong, Barnes, & Glantz, 2007).

Governance of political alliances has often been likened to herding cats. Each organization has its own political agenda, and your issue may not be as important to each of them as it is to you. At a minimum, have each organization agree in writing to work to achieve the alliance's goal, and to commit lobbying and grassroots advocacy assets to it. Voting power overall should be divided equally, which is a problem when one or a few organizations contribute the most money to the alliance. One option is to give greater weight to the voice of the moneyed partner in the manner in which that money is spent. More often than not, the most money is spent on paid media, so give the big contributor more voice in how the media campaign is conducted. To maintain the highest level of solidarity, each member of the alliance must feel like an equal partner in the endeavor; equality is in the mind of the beholder, so be sensitive to signs of discontent and deal with it. A fracture or collapse of an alliance at a critical point in the advocacy campaign can be a disaster.

Strong alliance leadership is another challenge. Not all members will commit personnel for the day-to-day operations of the alliance, but someone must take on the task. Look for one or more people who are passionate about the issue and willing to commit the time necessary to lead the group. An Executive Committee should be selected with an eye on those individuals with the most *political* experience, as the Executive Committee will be making decisions on the fly when your advocacy campaign is in the thick of the political battle. To guide the Executive Committee, all alliance members should sign a deal breaker agreement setting the minimum they will accept in the give-and-take of an advocacy battle (Americans for Nonsmokers' Rights, 2009).

Maintaining alliance cohesion and commitment through a long advocacy campaign can be difficult. There is a tendency to let internal communications shrink to fit the nucleus of organizations heavily involved in day-to-day matters to the exclusion of those not so heavily involved. Regular communications with *all* alliance partners is very important; it makes everyone feel like a part of the alliance and helps keep them energized. When you need to activate the grassroots advocates, having all alliance partners fully informed on campaign progress is vital.

The Effective Alliance Infrastructure

An important strength of the alliance comes from its ability to integrate members' lobbying capacities to work during periods in which the policymaking body is in session. State legislatures usually meet for only part of the year (see Chapter 4 for more details), but most municipality legislative bodies work year-round. The lobbying integration should be a formal one, with regular meetings for lobbyists to exchange information and share assignments.

Concomitant with this integration is adopting a protocol for interlinking the grassroots advocacy networks of all alliance members. Grassroots advocacy is the process of encouraging individual voters to contact their elected representatives in support of a policy initiative, and, when used properly (Moseley, Melton, & Francisco, 2008; Peregrin, 2011; Roberts, 2006), can be significantly powerful (Bergan, 2009). There is guidance in the literature (Frattaroli, 2003; Hanson, 1992; Kotzer, Smyth, Gill, Rapstine, & Thomas, 2001) for organizing grassroots advocacy networks. It is not necessary to combine all of the advocacy networks into a single one, as many organizations take a strong proprietary interest in their lists of members and supporters; the alliance's grassroots coordinator must have access to each member's grassroots coordinator so that a single e-mail action alert can be sent simultaneously to all grassroots coordinators, who then immediately distribute it to each members' grassroots advocates. With this protocol in place, the alliance's grassroots coordinator can create a single action alert that can be distributed to hundreds or even thousands of grassroots advocates in a matter of minutes. At crucial times in an advocacy campaign, every minute can make a significant difference in the outcome.

EVIDENCE-BASED POLICY DESIGN

Using Scientific Research in Advocacy

Once the analysis of the status quo is complete, the next step is to gather the evidence to provide support for the efficacy of your proposed solution to the problem. These data are essential to making your case for change to voters and policymakers.

Just as in clinical practice, in advocacy, the best intervention is evidence-based. Identify researchers with the relevant credentials who will work with you, including presenting their own research to policymakers, along with conducting meta analyses and literature reviews of the existing literature. Assemble all of the existing literature on your problem. See if there is any unpublished research in the pipeline that bears on your problem, but could be presented to policymakers. You may need to design and execute a research project specifically for your policy goal. See Chapter 8 for more details on the use of research for advocacy. Be sure to examine data that your opponents will likely use, and be prepared to explain or rebut it. The century-long debate on health care reform shows how harsh the battle of data can become, and you must be prepared for it.

The challenge to proponents of public health and health policy change is putting the scientific evidence to support their proposal into a form and language that policymakers can understand (Bayer & Colgrove, 2002; Bero, Montini, Bryan-Jones, & Mangurian, 2001; Harris, Luke, Zuckerman, & Shelton, 2009; Young & Borland, 2011). By their very nature, the worlds of policymakers and scientists are vastly different (Figure 3.1) (Brownson, Royer, Ewing, & McBride, 2006; Fielding et al., 2002). policymakers' desire for current data is a challenge to scientists who value peer-reviewed publication as the gold standard for research validity. With the rigorous standards scientists use for data collection and analysis, the preparation of manuscripts for publication, and the peer review process, it typically takes years from the commencement of data collection to publication. policymakers will also want to know what will happen if your proposal is adopted and scientists are reluctant or unwilling to make such predictions. Advocates must bridge this gap by presenting objective, scientific data in a concise, understandable way that assuages the policymakers' desire for

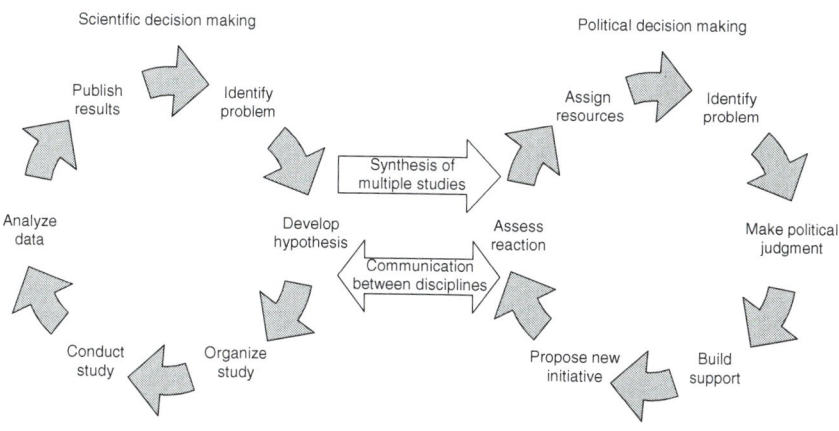

FIGURE 3.1
The "Real-World" Process of Decision Making in Science and Public Policy
Source: Reprinted from Brownson, R. et al. (2006). Researchers and policymakers: Travelers in parallel universes. *American Journal of Preventive Medicine, 30*(2), 164–172. With permission from Elsevier.

currency and prophecy; the best science takes time (meta analyses and literature reviews can often compress this time and present a broader base of relevant data), and the focus of the prophecy should be on what will likely happen if nothing is done, along with evidence showing how the proposed solution will affect the cause of the problem.

Policymakers are very often reluctant to deal with policy change that is new or novel, and will want to know if it has ever been tried before; research how other jurisdictions (domestic and foreign) have dealt with the problem (Nykiforuk, Eyles, & Campbell, 2008), but do so with the understanding that no two jurisdictions are alike (Bardach, 2012, p. 25, 26). This can also be a source of ideas for your policy change. Don't accept at face value the policy approach that other jurisdictions have adopted. How successful was the policy in dealing with the problem, and at what cost? Will it work in your jurisdiction? If you are proposing a policy change that has never been tried, research the literature for ideas from experts who are opining on the matter. If there is nothing to be found in other jurisdictions or the literature, you may have to use a pilot project to test your solution before pressing for the policy change; for example, consider a local ordinance before going for state legislation.

Once the research is completed, create a binder that can later be duplicated for sharing with policymakers and their staff, newspaper reporters and editorial boards, and executive department staff. You will be able to show that you are proposing an evidence-based solution to the cause of a real problem.

Designing the New Policy

If your problem has a single cause, policy design is a matter of looking at all available alternative solutions. If your problem has more than one cause, such as a large population of uninsured persons, you should select from among them which one you want to act upon. You can eat a whale only one bite at a time.

There are three basic goals of policy change: Eliminate the problem, alleviate it, or keep it from getting worse. Few problems lend themselves to a single solution, and it is important in designing a policy to examine all of the alternatives and then evaluate each. If there are several different policy approaches, compare and contrast them, perhaps picking the best features and combining them into a new synthesized approach, while avoiding any policy failures that may have occurred in other jurisdictions.

Public policy usually involves a delivery of benefits, an imposition of burdens, or a combination of both, through all types of coercive and persuasive methods called policy tools or instruments (Salamon, 2002).

A policy tool or instrument is a method through which governments seek a policy goal, such as a new law (Salamon & Lund, 1989). Familiar tools are criminal laws and coercive antipollution laws. Examples of persuasion are tax credits and deductions, grants, loans, and loan guarantees that encourage all manners of behavior. An example of a hybrid of both is the tradable permits proposed to limit total emissions of greenhouse gases to a maximum allowable annual level for all generators of greenhouse gases, in lieu of imposing restrictions on individual generators of greenhouse gases. Modern policy instruments often include complex methodologies of both coercion and persuasion to deal with complex problems.

Before beginning the design process, you must decide which venue you will be operating in: Legislation, administrative rulemaking, executive order, or litigation. There are a number of issues to consider in choosing the venue (Pralle, 2003), starting from the legal analysis of the current policy environment that you did earlier, which may show that there are several policy instruments that you could use, and that more than one approach is available. Is a new law needed? If there is an existing policy instrument that is not adequately addressing your problem, could new or amended regulations be a viable solution? The process of administrative rulemaking is usually less affected by political pressure and compromises than is legislation, and administrative regulations are usually less time consuming to change. Since the issuance of regulations is based on a legislative grant of authority, is the statutory authority sufficiently broad to permit the regulations you desire? If not, legislative change will be necessary first. Are there existing regulations that are not being implemented or enforced that cause or exacerbate your problem? Perhaps litigation could force the agency to act (described in Chapter 7). This analysis also leads you to the venue in which your advocacy will unfold.

Once you have determined what venue you will use to address your problem, you need to understand how that venue operates. Legislatures function under rules adopted by the bodies, administrative agency procedures are governed by statutes, and local government procedures may be based on charter or ordinance. Legislative advocacy is much more than knowing how a bill becomes law (detailed in Chapter 4); it is about how the detailed procedural rules affect this process. Knowing those procedural rules allows you to use them at crucial times to overcome adverse events or outflank your opposition. Administrative procedures and laws provide the step-by-step process that administrative agencies must follow to adopt rules and regulations, and the agencies themselves usually adopt additional rules set out in agency publications that give more detail on how the agency carries out its rulemaking function.

In designing your policy instrument, you must clearly have in mind whose behavior it is supposed to change, and target the policy at them. The "target groups" or "target populations" are those who will receive the benefits or burdens of the policy (Sabatier, 2007, p. 95). You need to consider the perspectives of the target or target groups when designing the policy. Those receiving benefits are most likely to be concerned with how the benefit will actually affect their lives, while those being burdened look at the cost of the policy in monetary terms and in terms of the difficulty of complying with rules and regulations (Mazmanian & Sabatier, 1989, pp. 12–13).

Federal legislation, and to a lesser extent state legislation, sets out the broad parameters of policy, and leaves the crafting of implementing rules and regulations to the agency in charge of administration and enforcement. Early in the design process, determine if the governmental unit likely to be implementing the policy will be friendly or unfriendly to your proposal (Hicklin & Godwin, 2009). Consideration of implementation issues should be an integral part of policy design, as many challenges to implementation (Häggblom & Möller, 2009; Jaeger & Yan, 2009; Montini & Bero, 2008; Ross & Dovers, 2008) can be avoided by anticipating and dealing with them in the policy design phase (Mazmanian & Sabatier, 1989; Pressman & Wildavsky, 1984; Satterlund, Lee, Moore, & Antin, 2009). Policymakers heed the advice of administrative agencies, and you should work to gain agency support; it will also make implementation go much more smoothly. If you cannot get agency support, you will need to craft a strategy to overcome its opposition.

Today's complex problems often need complex solution schemes involving various stakeholders inside and outside of government (deLeon & Varda, 2009). It is wise to consult all other stakeholders who will be affected by your policy, including your opponents. Knowing all stakeholders' perspectives will assist you in your policy design. Once opponents understand how and why the problem must be dealt with, their opposition may wane. You may be able to assuage or accommodate the concerns of your opponents in a way that will eliminate their opposition without compromising the attainment of your policy goal. Even if you cannot accommodate the opposition, you will have a clearer understanding of the bases of the opposition and can fashion a better rebuttal to the opposition's arguments in fighting for your proposal and its implementation.

Once you have settled on potential solutions, it is a good idea to test those alternatives through more voter polling. There are two areas that need to be polled: Does the public agree that the problem is important and needs to be addressed? Also, from among alternative solutions, which have the highest levels of support? The polling data on alternative solutions allows you to refine the solution and frame your message before going public with it, and policymakers want to know how their constituents stand on a problem and its solution.

In finally determining which of the alternative courses of action to pursue, there are a number of criteria that could be applied (Bardach, 2012, pp. 31–47). Among the most common are efficiency and efficacy. Others are equity and justice. The most vexatious is political acceptability; can we get it adopted?

In considering political acceptability, advocates have to balance how much, if anything, they are willing to give up to get the policy adopted against what is efficient, efficacious, equitable, just, and all of the other criteria they have attached to the policy goal. While compromise is inevitable in politics, be careful of the trap of thinking that "half a loaf is better than no loaf." It is often difficult to get the rest of the loaf later, when policymakers have seen that you are willing to take only half a loaf. You may be better served to hold out for the whole loaf and use your educational campaign to increase public awareness of the need to fix the problem (which improves your polling numbers), educate the policymakers, and wear down the opposition. Successful policy advocacy can take time, so be patient but persistent.

THE STRATEGIC PLAN

The strategic plan is largely driven by a timetable for action, the venue you choose, and the likely opponents you will face.

A Timetable for Action

When a problem is identified by activists, the reaction is to fix it "now." When that fix involves changing public policy, the "now" can be a decade. A timetable brings realism to the process. A preliminary timetable should be created very early in the process to set deadlines for commencement and completion of each of the components of the advocacy campaign.

Some of the key timetable components can be carried out simultaneously. For example, alliance building should start as soon as the problem is defined. If the initial polling research on voter issue awareness shows weak awareness or concern, a basic media awareness campaign should be started concurrently.

The Policy Venue

Legislation takes place at the federal, state, and local levels. Regardless of the level in which you are operating, advancing a legislative policy instrument requires educating individual legislators and their staff.

Elected officials come and go, but legislative staffers are usually career employees of the legislative body. It is helpful to identify legislative staff members who regularly work on your problem area or similar problem areas, as they are likely to be experts and just need your data to understand what you propose. Legislative staffers have considerable influence on legislators because they are trusted, reliable sources of relevant information.

Administrative rulemaking takes place in an executive branch agency (such as the Federal Department of Health and Human Services or the State Department of Health) that is already an expert in dealing with the broad category of problems like yours. As with legislative staffers, agency staff also need your data on what is causing the problem and data on your proposed solution (Bero et al., 2001).

Understanding and Combating the Opposition

Your obvious opponents will be those whose interests will be negatively affected if your policy proposal is adopted. In many cases, even a slight negative affect is enough to awaken the opposition, which fears the "slippery slope" effect of a small first step leading to a chain of related events culminating in some significant effect (Rizzo & Whitman, 2003). Your opponents may also hide behind third-party allies to enhance the legitimacy of the opposition campaign (Dearlove, Bialous, & Glantz, 2002; Mandel & Glantz, 2004; Ritch & Begay, 2001). Some opponents with no interest that will be negatively affected by your policy proposal will nevertheless oppose you on ideological grounds; for example, libertarians who oppose most government intrusion in individuals' decisions.

Understanding *who* your opponents are is just the first step; you also need to understand *how* they will oppose you. Unless your problem is unique and has never been addressed before in any jurisdiction, look at how the opposition acted in other jurisdictions. Contact organizations in those other jurisdictions with experience in working on issues similar to yours. News media coverage on important policy issues is a rich source of public statements of proponents and opponents and analyses of issues. Official reports of legislative committee hearings, available as transcripts and audio files, can give you actual examples of facts presented and arguments made by opposition representatives. Corporations often reveal in annual reports how they are dealing, or plan to deal, with issues that could affect profits. Also look at trade association journals and newsletters of the industry that will be an opponent, along with the trade journals and newsletters of their usual allies.

EXECUTING THE STRATEGIC PLAN

Identify Potential Policymaker Champions

For legislation, you will want to recruit one or more members of the policymaking body to sponsor your policy instrument. Look for members with an interest in health, health care, or public health. Discuss the problem and proposed solutions with them to get their feedback. Beware of policymakers who say they support the idea, but are not really committed to it. Your issue can get lost among other issues in which the policymaker is more interested and invested. You will want a committed champion with whom you can work closely. Working with this champion, identify others in the policymaking body who may be potential supporters of your measure. The more groundwork you can lay before launching the campaign, the more effort you will save later in mustering the votes needed to adopt your policy instrument.

Draft the Policy Instrument

A legislative policy instrument should be drafted with assistance from lawyers. Staff of the policymaking body who are charged with such drafting can also be very helpful. You will want to be intimately involved in the drafting so that the instrument is what you want the policymaking body to adopt.

Administrative agencies are often very territorial about rulemaking. It may help if you present a draft of what you want in order to expedite the process, and then offer to assist in further work on the regulations—especially if you can provide expertise that the agency can use. Since the rulemaking will involve public notice of proposed new regulations and a public comment period, you should also provide comment in this formal part of the process.

Getting and Keeping the Public on Your Side

Policymakers respond to constituents, and you need an early start to the process of getting support from the public. The goal is to elevate the problem to the policymaking agenda where policymakers will deal with it (Birkland, 2011, pp. 170–172; Mebane & Blendon, 2001). An advocacy campaign can span years, so early education of the public about the problem you are seeking to solve is essential; you can ease the public into your proposed solution later, after the public understands the importance of policy change. The media (see Chapter 5) is used for three fundamental purposes: Educating the public and policymakers, grassroots advocacy to reach policymakers through Letters to the Editor or op-ed pieces, and as an agenda-setting tool.

You can measure how well you have educated the public through voter opinion polling. The educational process can take longer than expected, so do the polling at regular intervals until you have a substantial majority of the public agreeing that the problem is important and needs to be addressed. You may lose some support when you go public with your proposed solution (Lum, Barnes, & Glantz, 2009). With a high level of support, you can press the policymakers to put the issue on the agenda (Mebane & Blendon, 2001).

In addition to educating the public on the issue, the media is a powerful public policy agenda-setting force (Kingdon, 2011, pp. 57–61) to move an issue onto the decision-making agenda (Birkland, 2011, pp. 44–54). Here your task is to educate the media about the importance of the issue and the need for policymakers to address it. Start by working with news writers and reporters who cover the issue. Give them the research notebook so that stories about the issue are properly framed and supported by the evidence. Get to know the Capitol Bureau reporters; they work at the capitol, write about what is happening there, and can be great sources of ideas for putting your story in proper political context.

There are several ways to get your story in print or on the evening news, such as press releases, press conferences, and media events. Press releases should be used sparingly; they are impersonal. Press conferences give the media a chance to ask questions, giving your spokespersons an opportunity to clarify and explain. Media events, however, can be like performance art. Here you can bring your experts and victims of the problem together, to put a real face on the problem. They can also be used to address the arguments raised by your opponents that your solution will impose unacceptable burdens on them as stakeholders required to engage or prohibited from engaging in the behavior you are trying to modify. It is rare that your proposed solution will be opposed by all such stakeholders; some will see it as acceptable, balanced out by a benefit, or as a positive for them. Find those who support what you are trying to do and are willing to speak out in person and on the record; it can be a powerful rebuttal to the opposition.

Perhaps the most important aspect of the media as agenda-setters is the editorial page. If you are successful in getting your story out and in building public interest in the issue, editorial boards will likely consider taking a position on it. Editorials help shape public support (or opposition) for important policy issues, and they inform policymakers about how important the issue is. To significantly increase your chances of having that position taken on your side, you need to take your research book directly to the editorial boards of newspapers while you are working with the news writers and reporters. Editorial boards are driven by facts, and you want to present the facts framed your way; bring your most articulate expert so that questions can be answered. It may take more than one visit with an editorial board to get it to act. Don't overlook the local newspapers in the districts of key policymakers, such as the leadership and key committee chairs in the legislature, as those legislators are sensitive to what their home town media are saying about policy issues.

Think of the media as one of your lobbyists, giving voice to your issue and your solution to the problem. Journalists strive to give balance to a news story, including your opponents' views. By giving journalists objective and reliable facts, expert opinions, victims' statements, testimonials of supportive stakeholders, and logical justification for your solution, the news stories will become an extension of your lobbying efforts.

Launching the Campaign

When is the right time to push your problem onto the agenda? This is always the vexing question. If public support is high, the media is giving the problem regular attention, and your alliance members are ready, the time is probably right (Mebane & Blendon, 2001). Draft your policy instrument, find a champion or two from among the members of the policymaking body to sponsor your policy instrument, do final voter polling to show the level of voter support for your proposed solution, and go for it.

Swaying the Policymakers

You can communicate with policymakers in different ways, depending on the venue. Legislators should get both emotional and factual information: For example, how does the problem affect the legislator's constituents, why will your proposed solution change that affect for the better, and what is the cost of inaction versus the cost of your proposed solution? Emotional information can best be presented by and about constituents whose lives are affected by the problem. Factual information is presented by experts on the problem who can explain how the problem can be solved, discuss the cost of inaction versus the cost of the proposed solution, and answer policymakers' questions.

Legislative policymakers want to know how their constituents stand on the issue, and they learn that from many sources. Share your best voter polling data with them. Public opinion influences public policy, often strongly (Burstein, 2003), and is especially important in offsetting powerful special interests in health policymaking (Turner, O'Connor, & Rademacher, 2009). Some legislators do their own polling of constituents through newsletters or questionnaires. They read the Letters to the Editor in the local newspaper, a useful tool for your grassroots advocacy campaign. Grassroots advocacy also involves constituents contacting their legislators by face-to-face meetings, letters, e-mails, and telephone calls, the kind of very effective grassroots advocacy that you must initiate. Another group of potentially important allies are "grasstops" advocates, elected officials at a lower level of government, who are viewed by legislators as spokespersons for their constituents; this group is particularly important when the problem you are seeking to solve adversely affects those lower levels of government.

Administrative agencies need factual, evidence-based information to guide their rulemaking, which must be based on existing law. Agencies must be convinced that a change in existing rules and regulations is necessary to carry out the intent of that existing law, to correct an inadequacy in its implementation, address a new issue within the scope of that existing law, or whatever is causing the problem that can be fixed by rulemaking.

One policymaker all too often overlooked in an advocacy campaign is the executive branch head (president, governor, or mayor), who usually has the power to veto the measure you have worked so hard to get passed. Here your task is to identify the staff member or members who are assigned to working on legislative matters and to educate them in the same way you educate legislators, editorial boards, and voters, and to do so at the same time. It is too late to start this process after the measure is passed; you need to know as early as possible what the chief executive will do, as it may shape how you fashion the measure.

Key players in swaying policymakers are lobbyists. This is particularly true on medical and public health issues, where the lobbyists are viewed by legislators as credible and useful sources of information (Cohen et al., 1997). There is another very important reason for using lobbyists—their presence at the seat of policymaking on a daily basis while your victims of the problem, experts, and grassroots and grasstops advocates make an appearance and then go home. Legislation is passed in phases, with short-term flurries of activity on a given bill followed by long periods of dead zone. The lobbyists are there during these dead zones, engaged in regular and repeated contact with the legislators to keep your issue in their view, to answer questions, and to be your eyes and ears for intelligence on what the opposition is doing. A good lobbyist is the glue that holds all of your other advocacy efforts together.

The army of grassroots advocates supporting your alliance members is the most powerful weapon you and your lobbyists have to sway the policymakers to vote your way. A good lobbyist is a field commander in the heat of battle with a minute-to-minute view of what is going on and what is needed to win the day. Often what is needed to win the day is grassroots advocates reacting quickly to Action Alerts originated by your lobbyist to contact their personal legislators by phone, e-mail, or fax. Response time for many Action Alerts is measured in hours, not days; many an advocacy effort has faltered or failed because grassroots advocates were not properly used.

POLICY IMPLEMENTATION AND EVALUATION

In some cases, getting legislation passed is the easy part; now you may have to deal with implementing rules or regulations promulgated by the agency designated to effectuate the new law. If you designed your policy instrument correctly, with implementation issues clearly in mind, crafting rules or regulations should go smoothly. To be sure that implementation accords with the intent of the policy design, you should be actively involved in the rulemaking process.

Too many advocates think that once the policy becomes law and is implemented, their job is done. Policies do not exist in a vacuum. Implementation may be adversely affected by the way agency managers view the policy (Hicklin & Godwin, 2009). Over time, circumstances change and the policy may no longer work. There is also the Law of Unintended Consequences (Merton, 1936), under which the policy outcomes are different from what was intended. Policy evaluation is a key component of advocacy success, and is important even in times of budget constraints (Bozeman & Massey, 1982).

Policy evaluation has become an established field of study by academics (Rossi, Lipsey, & Freeman, 2004) and the literature is replete with studies of health policy evaluations (Adeyanju, 1991; Farmer & Currie, 2009; Fong et al., 2006; Harris et al., 2010; Mendoza, Watson, & Cullen, 2010). When you plan your evaluation, give the new policy time to fully develop before embarking on the evaluation because you want to look at not only the operational aspects of the new policy, but also whether the policy achieved its intended goal or goals. If problems are found, start a new advocacy cycle to fix the problems.

REFLECTION QUESTIONS

1. Why have I avoided involvement in policy advocacy?
2. Where in the advocacy process do I see myself acting?
3. What went wrong in a failed advocacy campaign that I know about?

PRACTICE MAKES PERFECT

1. Write a "problem definition" on an issue that you are interested in.
2. Make a list of potential alliance partners to work on that problem.
3. Create a slogan for the advocacy campaign on that problem.

REFERENCES

Adeyanju, M. (1991). Public knowledge, attitudes, and behavior toward Kansas mandatory seatbelt use: Implications for public health policy. *Journal of Health & Social Policy, 3*(2), 117–135.

Affholter, D. (1994). Outcome monitoring. In J. Wholey, H. Hatry, & K. Newcomer (Eds.), *Handbook of practical program evaluation*. San Francisco, CA: Jossey Bass.

Americans for Nonsmokers' Rights. (2009). *Determining your dealbreakers*. Retrieved from www.no-smoke.org/pdf/dealbreakers.pdf

Anderson, G. (1992). The courts and health policy: Strengths and limitations. *Health Affairs (Millwood), 11*(4), 95–110.

Bardach, E. (2012). *A practical guide for policy analysis: The eightfold path to more effective problem solving* (4th ed.). Washington, DC: CQ Press.

Barnes, R. (2002). The Oklahoma alliance on health or tobacco. A partnership for a healthier Oklahoma. *Journal of the Oklahoma State Medical Association, 95*(3), 126.

Bayer, R., & Colgrove, J. (2002). Science, politics, and ideology in the campaign against environmental tobacco smoke. *American Journal of Public Health, 93*(6), 949–954.

Bergan, D. (2009). Does grassroots lobbying work? *American Politics Research, 37*(2), 327–352.

Bero, L., Montini, T., Bryan-Jones, K., & Mangurian, C. (2001). Science in regulatory policy making: Case studies in the development of workplace smoking restrictions. *Tobacco Control, 10*(4), 329–336.

Birkland, T. A. (2011). *Introduction to the policy process* (3rd ed.). Armonk, NY: M.E. Sharpe.

Bozeman, B., & Massey, J. (1982). Investing in policy evaluation: Some guidelines for skeptical public managers. *Public Administration Review, 42*(3), 264–270.

Bozlak, C., & Kelley, M. (2009). Youth participation in a community campaign to pass a clean indoor air ordinance. *Health Promotion Practice, 11*(4), 530–540.

Brownson, R., Royer, C., Ewing, R., & McBride, T. (2006). Researchers and policymakers travelers in parallel universes. *American Journal of Preventive Medicine, 30*(2), 164–172.

Burstein, P. (2003). The impact of public opinion on public policy: A review and an agenda. *Political Science Quarterly, 56*(1), 29–40.

Cohen, J., Goldstein, A., Flynn, B., Munger, M., Gottlieb, N., Solomon, L., ... Munger, M. C. (1997). State legislators' perceptions of lobbyists and lobbying on tobacco control issues. *Tobacco Control, 6*, 332–336.

Dearlove, J. V., Bialous, S. A., & Glantz, S. A. (2002). Tobacco industry manipulation of the hospitality industry to maintain smoking in public places. *Tobacco Control, 11*(2), 94–104.

deLeon, P., & Varda, D. (2009). Toward a theory of collaborative policy networks: Identifying structural tendencies. *The Policy Studies Journal, 37*(1), 59–74.

Farmer, J., & Currie, M. (2009). Evaluating the outcomes of rural health policy. *Australian Journal of Rural Health, 17*, 53–57.

Fielding, J., Marks, J., Myers, B., Nolan, P., Rawson, R., & Toomey, K. (2002). How do we translate science into public health policy and law? *Journal of Law, Medicine & Ethics, 30*, 22–32.

Fong, G., Cummings, K. M., Borland, R., Hastings, G., Hyland, A., Giovino, G., . . . Thompson, M. E. (2006). The conceptual framework of the International Tobacco Control (ITC) Policy Evaluation Project. *Tobacco Control, 15*(Suppl. III), iii3–iii11.

Frattaroli, S. (2003). Grassroots advocacy for gun violence prevention: A status report on mobilizing a movement. *Journal of Public Health Policy, 24*(3), 332–354.

Gruen, R., Campbell, E., & Blumenthal, D. (2006). Public roles of US physicians: Community participation, political involvement, and collective advocacy. *Journal of the American Medical Association, 296*(20), 2467–2475.

Häggblom, A., & Möller, A. (2009). Implementation of a government policy programme on Operation Kvinnofrid. *Nursing Inquiry, 16*(1), 43–52.

Hanson, C. (1992). System-directed grassroots advocacy. *Health Progress, 73*(3), 52–53, 65.

Harris, C., Bradlyn, A., Tompkins, N., Purkey, M., Kennedy, K., & Kelley, G. (2010). Evaluating the West Virginia health lifestyles act: Methods and procedures. *Journal of Physical Activity and Health, 7*(Suppl. 1), S31–S39.

Harris, J., Luke, D., Zuckerman, R., & Shelton, S. (2009). Forty years of secondhand smoke research: The gap between discovery and delivery. *American Journal of Preventive Medicine, 36*(6), 538–548.

Hicklin, A., & Godwin, E. (2009). Agents of change: The role of managers in public policy. *Policy Studies Journal, 37*(1), 13–20.

Hong, M.-K., Barnes, R., & Glantz, S. (2007). *Tobacco control in California 2003–2007: A missed opportunity*. San Francisco, CA: Center for Tobacco Control Research and Education, University of California. Retrieved from http://repositories.cdlib.org/ctcre/tcpmus/CA2007

Jaeger, P., & Yan, Z. (2009). One law with two outcomes: Comparing the implementation of CIPA in public libraries and schools. *Information Technology and Libraries, 28*(1), 6–14.

Kingdon, J. (2011). *Agendas, alternatives, and public policies* (2nd ed.). Chicago, IL: Pearson Education, Inc.

Kotzer, A., Smyth, M., Gill, A., Rapstine, T., & Thomas, L. (2001). Grassroots advocacy in action: Successes and opportunities for pediatric nurses. *Journal of the Society of Pediatric Nurses, 6*(1), 39–41.

Lee, P., Oliver, T., Benjamin, A., & Lee, D. (2006). Politics, health policy, and the American character. *Stanford Law and Policy Review, 17*, 7–32.

Lum, K., Barnes, R., & Glantz, S. (2009). Enacting tobacco taxes by direct popular vote in the United States: Lessons from 20 years of experience. *Tobacco Control, 18*, 377–386.

Mandel, L. L., & Glantz, S. A. (2004). Hedging their bets: Tobacco and gambling industries work against smoke-free policies. *Tobacco Control, 13*(3), 268–276.

Mazmanian, D., & Sabatier, P. (1989). *Implementation and public policy*. Lanham, MD: University Press of America.

Mebane, F., & Blendon, R. (2001). Political strategy 101: How to make health policy and influence political people. *Journal of Child Neurology, 16*(7), 513–519.

Mendoza, J., Watson, K., & Cullen, K. (2010). Change in dietary energy density after implementation of the Texas public school nutrition policy. *Journal of the American Dietetic Association, 110,* 434–440.

Merton, R. (1936). The unanticipated consequences of purposive social action. *American Sociological Review, 1*(6), 894–904.

Montini, T., & Bero, L. (2008). Implementation of a workplace smoking ban in bars: The limits of local discretion. *BMC Public Health, 8,* 402–414.

Moseley, C., Melton, L., & Francisco, V. (2008). Grassroots advocacy campaign for HIV/AIDS prevention: Lessons from the field. *Health Promotion Practice, 9*(3), 253–261.

Nykiforuk, C., Eyles, J., & Campbell, H. (2008). Smoke-free spaces over time: A policy diffusion study of bylaw development in Alberta and Ontario, Canada. *Health & Social Care in the Community, 16*(1), 64–74.

Oliver, T. (2006). The politics of public health policy. *Annual Review of Public Health, 27,* 195–233.

Peregrin, T. (2011). Helping grassroots advocacy efforts take root. *Journal of the American Dietetic Association, 111*(3), 356–358.

Pralle, S. (2003). Venue shopping, political strategy, and policy change: The internationalization of Canadian forest advocacy. *Journal of Public Policy, 23*(3), 233–260.

Pressman, J., & Wildavsky, A. (1984). *Implementation: How great expectations in Washington are dashed in Oakland* (3rd ed.). Berkeley, CA: University of California Press.

Quadango, J. (2005). *One nation uninsured: Why the U.S. has no national health insurance.* New York, NY: Oxford University Press.

Ritch, W. A., & Begay, M. E. (2001). Strange bedfellows: The history of collaboration between the Massachusetts restaurant association and the tobacco industry. *American Journal of Public Health, 91*(4), 598–603.

Rizzo, M., & Whitman, D. (2003). The camel's nose in in the tent: Rules, theories, and slippery slopes. *UCLA Law Review, 51*(2), 539–592.

Roberts, A. (2006). "All politics is local": The importance of grassroots advocacy. *Bulletin of the American College of Surgeons, 91(10),* 16–18.

Ross, A., & Dovers, S. (2008). Making the harder yards: Environmental policy integration in Australia. *Australian Journal of Public Administration, 67*(3), 245–260.

Rossi, P., Lipsey, M., & Freeman, H. (2004). *Evaluation: A systematic approach* (7th ed.). Thousand Oaks, CA: Sage Publications, Inc.

Sabatier, P. (Ed.). (2007). *Theories of the policy process* (2nd ed.). Boulder, CO: Westview Press.

Salamon, L. (Ed.). (2002). *The tools of government: A guide to the new governance.* New York, NY: Oxford University Press.

Salamon, L., & Lund, M. (1989). The tools approach: Basic analytics. In L. Salamon (Ed.), *Beyond privatization: The tools of government action.* Washington, DC: Urban Institute Press.

Satterlund, T., Lee, J., Moore, R., & Antin, T. (2009). Challenges to implementing and enforcing California's Smoke-Free Workplace Act in bars. *Drugs: Education, Prevention & Policy, 16*(5), 422–435.

Sherraden, M., Slosar, B., & Sherraden, M. (2002). Innovation in social policy: Collaborative policy advocacy. *Social Work, 47*(3), 209–221.

Stone, D. (1989). Causal stories and the formation of policy agendas. *Political Science Quarterly, 104*(2), 281–300.

Stone, D. (2002). *Policy paradox: The art of political decision making* (Ch. 8, Rev. ed.). New York, NY: W.W. Norton & Co.

Turner, S., O'Connor, P., & Rademacher, E. (2009). Inform, influence, evaluate: The power of state public opinion polls. *Health Affairs, 28*(1), 273–276.

Young, D., & Borland, R. (2011). Conceptual challenges in the translation of research into practice: It's not just a matter of "communication." *Translational Behavioral Medicine, 1*(2), 256–269.

4

Legislative Advocacy: Putting Your House in Order

KRISTIN KROEGER PTAKOWSKI

Advocacy is about opening doors and making friends to get your message across. If you are not at the table, you are on the menu!—Author unknown

This chapter will provide an overview of how legislative advocacy works and how you can make a difference for your practice and your patients.

For many people, especially health and mental health care professionals, being an advocate seems like a daunting task, and you may not know where to start. It is a world that you may not understand or that you just do not have time for. Your state capitol, or Washington, DC, is so far away. Can you really make a difference? You can!

As a clinician, you advocate daily for your patients—with insurance companies, pharmacy management companies, schools, and other social agencies. We often forget that advocacy is our first amendment right as U.S. citizens. We elect our legislators who are accountable to us, and we can petition them for redress of grievances. Advocacy is the act of pleading or arguing in favor of something, such as a cause, idea, or policy. It is about opening doors and making friends to get *your* message across. So, why advocate? Change does not just happen. Whether it is a bill that provides funding for new research protocols or one that regulates health care delivery, change such as this is driven by people and organizations committed to making a difference and who help to persuade others in the process. If you do not advocate, someone else will and you may not like the outcome.

There are multiple opportunities to influence change in a legislative process. Throughout this chapter we will explore how a bill becomes a law and the opportunities you have for change along the way. As you get involved in advocacy, it is important that you keep three things in mind:

- Policy change does not happen overnight; it takes time, sometimes a lot of time. It took more than a decade to get mental health parity passed through Congress.
- Be persistent. Keep communicating your message, time and time again. Do not be afraid to keep going at it until the right person listens to you, even though it may feel repetitive and frustrating at times. A new congress begins every 2 years and state sessions typically begin every year, so there will be new faces and priorities.
- Finally, compromise is inevitable. There is something called the "80% rule." Wyoming Senator Mike Enzi once said that Congress can get more done by focusing on the 80% on which they can agree (*Associated Press*, 2008). It is counterproductive to fall on the sword for that 20% on which you do not agree. There will always be chances to improve upon what you have. An example of this is the passage of mental health parity legislation (Domenici and Wellstone) in 2008. The issue of equality in health care costs for mental and physical illnesses had been debated for decades prior to its passing. In the mid-1990s, advocates tried for the passage of full parity but did not have the votes needed. In the end, Congress passed legislation that would end the lifetime and annual limits for mental illnesses. With persistence and consistent education about mental illnesses, and the need for cost effective and nondiscriminatory treatment, the mental health parity bill was passed 10 years later.

HOW A BILL BECOMES A LAW

It is important to know that at the federal level the congressional session covers 2 years, and in most states, legislatures start a new session each year. States vary with regard to the calendar term for their legislature; some terms run for 12 months and some for fewer. Five states—Montana, Nevada, North Dakota, Oregon, and Texas—are on a biennial schedule and hold a regular session every other year. In some states, the governor or legislature may call a special session that focuses on specific topics or issues. Keep in mind that if a bill is not passed within the legislative session of a congress, it will need to be reintroduced in the next congress. The slate is essentially wiped clean. Federal and all but one state legislature have two legislative chambers consisting of the House (also called the Assembly or House of Delegates in a few states) and Senate. Nebraska has a unicameral chamber called the legislature. Nebraska's Legislature is also the only state legislature in the United States that is nonpartisan. The senators are elected with no party affiliation next to their names on

4 Legislative Advocacy: Putting Your House in Order 53

the ballot, and the speaker and committee chairs are chosen at large so that members of any party can be chosen for these positions. Your federal senators are elected for a term of 6 years and your House members (called representatives or congressmen) are elected for 2-year terms. Members of the state senate generally serve four terms while House members are elected for 2 years. Bills can be introduced in either chamber; however, a bill must eventually pass both houses to become law. The exception to this is that bills for raising revenue must originate in the House, and never in the Senate.

So how do legislators decide what bills they want to champion? Many focus on issues that are close to them, their families and their friends. For instance, you will likely find that champions of children's mental health issues have a child, or know someone with a child, who suffers from mental illness. Another influence is the values of their constituents. For example, a senator from a large farming state is likely to focus more on agriculture subsidies than a senator from a state with less farming interests. A senator with a pediatric hospital in his state will be very concerned with pediatric specialty issues. Finally, current events have a large impact on policy advances. For example, bullying in schools has gotten a lot of media attention recently and as a result many state legislatures and the U.S. Congress have numerous bills outlining anti-bullying initiatives. In the House, any member may introduce a bill, by dropping it into a box called a "hopper." In the Senate, a member may introduce a bill after being recognized by the presiding officer and announcing the bill's introduction. When a senator or representative introduces a bill, it is sent to the clerk of the House or Senate, who gives it a number (starting with H.R. for the House and S. for the Senate) and title. The clerk will do a "first reading" in whichever chamber the bill originated, and then refer it to the proper committee(s) or subcommittee. The bill may be referred to more than one committee if provisions in the bill cross the jurisdiction of multiple committees. At this time, all members of the House or Senate are asked to cosponsor it. Cosponsoring is a way to show support. A committee may choose to act on the legislation or may leave it "in waiting," which essentially kills the bill.

If the bill shows significant support or is important to the committee chair or chamber leadership, it will likely get a hearing, for which witnesses are called to testify to support or oppose the legislation. This is one part of legislative advocacy for which establishing relationships with your elected officials and their offices is key, as you may therefore have the opportunity to testify. In most state legislatures, anyone is welcome to provide public testimony. These hearings often come up with short notice and your elected official's prior knowledge of you and your interests helps keep you in the loop. If you cannot testify in person, you also have the opportunity to submit written testimony to the committee. During the hearing the members of the committee will ask questions of the witnesses. If you want a specific issue to be discussed or emphasized at the hearing, you may ask your Representative if they will ask that question during the hearing. For example, if the chief executive officer of a teaching hospital is testifying about the need for increased graduate medical education funding, you might ask your legislator to ask him where, specifically, he would recommend investing new dollars. If the bill has support within the subcommittee or committee it will be "marked up." During a mark-up the bill is introduced and members of the committee can modify it with amendments. This is another opportunity for you to affect policy; if your member is on the committee, you may ask her to introduce an amendment. If a bill passes out of a subcommittee with a majority vote, it goes to the committee as a whole, again with the potential for amendments and another opportunity for you to recommend changes. After the bill clears the appropriate committee(s) it will be placed on the docket for a vote of the whole chamber. If the head of the chamber, such as the Speaker of the House or the Majority Leader in the Senate, decides that the bill will move forward for a floor debate, then the clerk reads the bill sentence by sentence, which is known as the second reading. Members may then debate the bill and offer amendments. This allows members who are not a part of the committee process to make changes to the bill. In the House of Representatives, the time for debate is limited by a cloture rule, which is a time limit for debate; but there is no such cloture restriction in the Senate, where 60 votes are required to end debate. This makes possible a filibuster, in which one or more opponents hold the floor to defeat the bill by never letting it come to a vote. The third reading consists of only the title of the bill and the bill is put to a vote, which may be by voice or roll call. A vote is often taken by roll call when one party wants a record of who voted for and against the bill. A voice vote does not allow anyone to find out after the vote how someone voted. Recorded votes are automatically held when the House is voting on an appropriations bill, a bill to raise taxes, or the annual budget resolution. If the bill receives a positive vote from one chamber it must have the same from the other chamber in order to move forward. Two identical bills, one in each chamber, are collectively referred to as companion legislation. In an ideal scenario, both bills pass out their respective committees in identical form, but this is not often the case. If the bills are not identical, a conference committee, comprised of the chairs and co-chairs of the committees to which it was previously referred and other members appointed by the leaders of both chambers, tries to work out the differences and send an agreed upon version back to both chambers for a final vote.

When a bill passes both chambers it goes to the chief executive, either the president or governor, for signature. At the federal level, the president may sign it or veto it. If the bill is vetoed, a two-thirds majority vote of the House and Senate are required to override the veto and pass the bill anyway. A similar procedure happens in state legislatures. However, the governor can opt to take no action on the bill, as a political maneuver, and in some states this inaction leads to the bill becoming law after a defined period of time. Figure 4.1 below graphically depicts the key elements of this legislative process as described above.

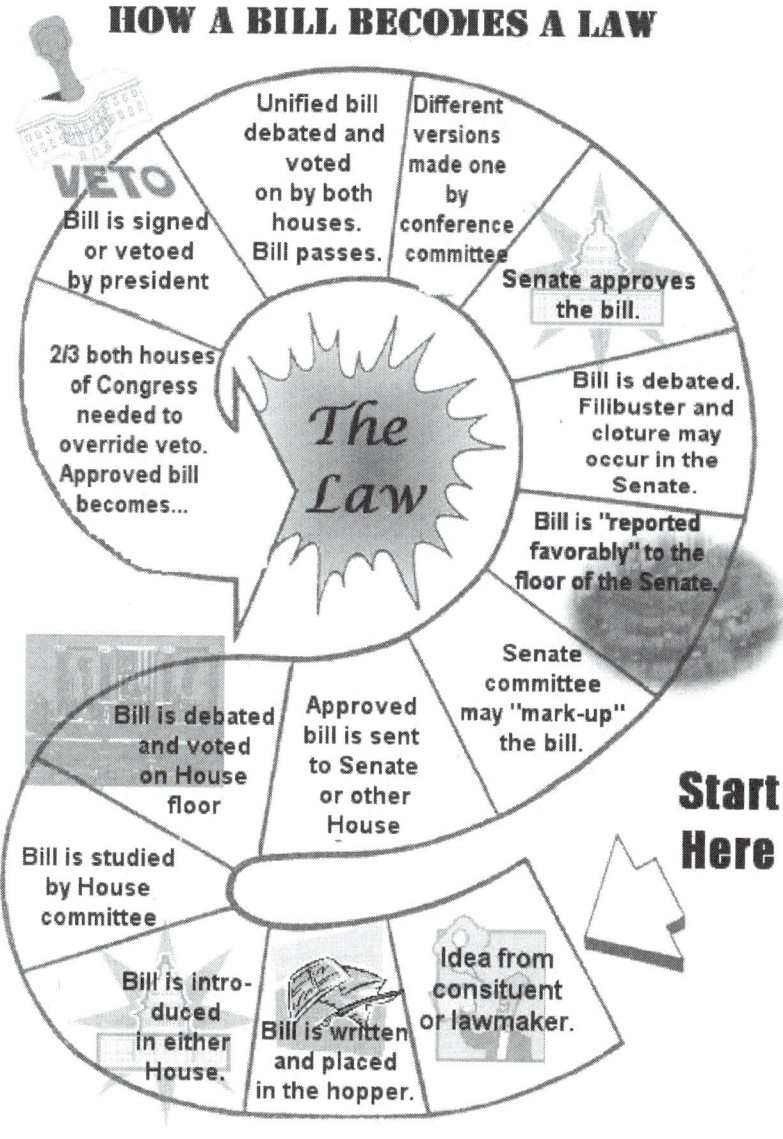

FIGURE 4.1
A Game Board Designed for Students That Depicts the Legislative Process.
Source: With permission from George Cassutto: http://www.cyberlearning-world.com/lessons/civics/lp.bill_to_law.htm

As you can probably tell, state and federal legislative processes are similar but with a few exceptions. However, advocating at the state level is often different. While your members of Congress often cover large districts and may seem quite distant from you, state legislators are often more approachable and likely live closer by. In most states, they often continue their professions and work as part-time legislators. As a result, they can see first hand many of the issues affecting the community. Most state legislators do not have the time or staff to research and hone their knowledge on every issue that comes before them. Due to the vast number of bills considered each year, legislators cannot become experts on every bill that crosses their desks. This is where health care professionals can be a valuable resource to them. Many of the issues that legislators face in this arena are highly specialized and technical. Legislators look for individuals with expertise in specific fields who can concisely articulate the complexities of an issue and the impact their votes could have on those they govern.

Finally, state legislation is a bit like gossip; it catches on pretty quickly in other states. This makes the legislative process easier in neighboring states, and it can also influence federal policy makers to take up an issue. Whether you are advocating at the state or federal levels, the advocacy skills are the same and you have many opportunities to make change. It takes persistence, relationship building, and teamwork to do so.

Understanding the basics of how the legislative process works is an important first step to being an advocate. Many professional organizations have offices that can assist health care professionals to determine where they can make a difference in the process.

ADVANCING YOUR CAUSE

No one can do it alone. That is why it is important to think through who might be potential allies in your advocacy efforts. Relationships play a key part in legislative advocacy. As clinicians, just as we build relationships with patients who build trust with us, as advocates we have to build relationships with our policy makers if we want to be effective. This is much easier at the state level than at the federal level. It is important to determine which legislators have supported your cause in the past. Do they have a particular personal interest, or if there is a specific need in their community or state? For example, former Senators Pete Domenici (NM) and Paul Wellstone (MN) each had a family member affected by mental illness and they were both strong champions for legislation to improve access to mental health services.

It is very important to demonstrate to policy makers that, as an advocate, you are representing many constituencies, institutions, and voters in their communities. The alliances of distinct partners who come together temporarily to take joint action are essential to advocacy. There are many different partners you could work with to advance your cause. Consider consumer advocacy groups, other professional groups such as medical colleagues, as well as other more specific organizations such as parent teacher organizations if you were advocating for a school-related cause. Building a coalition of partners allows smaller parties to increase their power.

Elected officials get thousands of letters a year and you may wonder whether your one letter would make any sort of difference. If you wrote that legislator a letter, a local pediatrician wrote her own letter saying something similar, and a parent wrote something similar, you are going to greatly increase your chances of being heard. The sum is definitely greater than the parts and it provides some political muscle.

Working with others in coalitions not only helps you save resources, because a group of people can do more than one person, but it also shows policy makers that there is consensus on an issue, and policy makers like consensus. It helps them feel more confident that they are receiving credible and complete information from experts on multiple sides of a particular issue. When building coalitions, it is important to keep a few things in mind, and they are basic tenets of relationship building:

- Mutual understanding: Each organization should respect its partners' mission, goals, and purpose.
- Develop some clearly defined goals and a specific plan of action to achieve them. Do not try to change the world—just try to change one piece of policy at a time.
- Appreciate each other's differences. Groups with varying viewpoints may not agree on all decisions and, again, that is okay.
- Be flexible. Allow each coalition partner to operate within its own organizational structure.

Lastly, coalitions are not permanent. While you may agree with other organizations on one particular issue, you may not share priorities in other policy areas, and that is okay. Organizations often come together in a coalition for a specific action, but do not necessarily work together on everything.

HOW TO COMMUNICATE YOUR MESSAGE

Once you have decided who will be your allies in your advocacy efforts, it is important to think about how you will communicate your message. First you should choose your communication based on what you want to accomplish. If you are just beginning the relationship-building process, choose a method that will get you some face time. But if there is an upcoming vote that you want to weigh in on, you may want to e-mail or call, not wait until you can schedule a meeting.

Face time with your elected official and/or staff is key to establishing relationships. Some think they have to meet with their legislator in person to make a difference. However, meeting with staff can be just as effective, or even more so. Whether it is in your home district, State office, or in Washington, DC, all offices are aware of who comes to talk with them and what they are concerned about. Staff members serve as the eyes and ears for their bosses, and if there is a constituent with a particular expertise that may help them with a policy issue, they usually know and may call on you for assistance. Everyone says it is important to know who your congressman is; even more important is that she/he knows who you are.

However, meeting with your Representative is just one type of advocacy—there are many more. They range from quick approaches, such as sending an e-mail or making a phone call, to approaches that are more involved, such as providing testimony, holding briefings, attending town hall meetings, and inviting legislators to an event or award ceremony. Letters, e-mails, and phone calls to an elected office is effective when a vote is pending. Before votes on high-profile issues, elected officials' offices can get flooded with phone calls and e-mails weighing in on both sides of the issue. This input helps officials know how their constituents want them to vote.

When elected officials are in session, educational briefings provide opportunities for legislators and their staff to gain a greater knowledge on a particular issue. Briefings are generally held by an organization or coalition and are sponsored by one or more members. Expert speakers are chosen to provide a balanced presentation about the topic under discussion. The briefing is often held to gain support for a piece of legislation. As mentioned earlier, one way to advocate during the bill-making process is to provide public comment in state legislators. Hearings are posted on the web a few days ahead of time and there is a time-limited, face-to-face public comment period. If you cannot make it to the state capitol, you also have the opportunity to submit your statement in writing. At the federal level there is no face-to-face public comment, but you may submit your comments, in writing to the committee.

During recess (between sessions) or on the weekends, many legislators will hold town hall meetings to address issues their constituents are concerned about. In addition to hearings mentioned above, town hall meetings are also an opportunity to ask your elected official a question about pending legislation or to recommend that he addresses an issue. These town hall gatherings often receive local and, sometimes, national media attention. Most recently, you may remember town hall meetings during the health care reform debate in 2009; more than two-thirds of

Americans (69%) closely followed news accounts of these town hall meetings (Newport, 2009). Organized rallies can also attract the attention of local officials and will raise awareness of your issues. This often brings additional media attention to your issue.

One of the best ways to advocate for your cause and educate elected officials is to invite them to an event you are holding and share your issue with them first hand. For example, if you are looking for support for a children's center, invite her/him to the center. Invite parents to talk with her/him about the benefits of the center for the children. Giving awards to legislators whom you supported on an action they took will also help to build stronger relationships. Often, legislators do not hear enough about what they are doing right and appreciate the recognition!

Whenever you contact a legislator's office, you should first and foremost identify yourself as a constituent. When communicating your message you want to quantify things as much as possible and have data to back it up. For example "only X% of children and adolescents in need of treatment for mental illness receive it. In our state, this means that there are Y number of children not receiving the services they need." To balance your data, be sure to tell your story or the stories of the families you work with and what the issue means to your practice. For example, if you are advocating for an increased workforce, share the typical wait time to get an appointment with you.

As you prepare to talk to a legislator about an issue, it is important to do your homework ahead of time. Have an understanding of how she or he has voted on similar issues in the past and be prepared to address the following questions.

- What are the merits of the issue?
- What impact does it have on the legislator's district?
- Does it involve possible job losses or gains?
- What is the cost?
- What is the issue's impact on the economy or business?
- Does the issue have the commitment of an interest group?
- Does the issue have support from the president or governor?
- What is the general sentiment about the issue?
- Try to think about the issue from a legislator's perspective and come prepared with some answers for their possible questions. Finally, be clear about what you want the legislator to do. Be as specific as possible, whether it is to vote no or yes on something, or cosponsor a bill.

With the internet, tracking legislation has become very easy. When bills are introduced they are given a number and there are numerous websites to track its programs. For federal legislation, sites such as THOMAS (http://thomas.loc.gov), Open Congress (www.opencongress.org), and

GovTrack (www.govtrack.us) can all help determine what committee the bill is referred to, how members voted, and who is on a related committee. It will also give you a summary of the bill and who has cosponsored it. These sites are also helpful if you are searching for bills related to your issues. They also provide a way to find out what types of bills have already been introduced and whether you can support these. State legislative tracking is usually accessed through your state government's website. On most state sites you can see summaries and full texts of the bills, as well as where the bill stands in the legislative process and upcoming public comment periods. Tracking multiple states' legislation is not free and will require a subscription to a larger database. StateNet and West Laws "WestClip" service or Lexis' "Eclipse" service can provide these services. However, many professional associations' government affairs offices track state legislation and your membership often allows you access to the service, or at least to frequent updates.

USING THE MEDIA FOR LEGISLATIVE ADVOCACY

As reviewed in greater detail in Chapter 5, the media is a great way to raise awareness about mental illness and treatment because it gets your message out to a wider audience. How does media advocacy relate to the legislative advocacy? Decisions to support legislative initiatives are frequently influenced by media coverage. Every congressional office has a staff person who monitors the news in your state and clip articles that mention your representative or senator by name. If you mention them in a letter to the editor or an opinion piece (i.e., an "op-ed," usually written by a person not on the paper's editorial board), their offices will take notice. So will other people in the state or district. And the more this publicity happens, the more likely a legislator is to act.

We all know that there is a lot of "spin" that goes on around any issue. Media advocacy can help counteract this sort of misinformation. When you as health and mental health professionals engage in this type of advocacy, you have an opportunity to break down the myths and fallacies and help the public understand the real story.

When you reach out to local media, you should keep your goal in mind; you are trying to influence policies and public opinions. When you first start doing media advocacy, you may not know exactly whom to approach. Do some research and know your target audience. Think about the best way to frame your message. Ask yourself, "Who reads that particular paper? Do they tend to have a more conservative or liberal stand on things?" Take this political landscape into account.

Also, find out who covers health issues for your local paper and reach out to them. You can usually find this on the publication's website, by following the paper regularly, or by calling its office. Once you find out who that reporter is, try to build a relationship and offer yourself as a resource to her. Many reporters are looking for locals who have a specific expertise. If they write something related to your issue, respond with a letter to the editor, or suggest an op-ed on the topic. Finally, pay attention to current events that may have piqued the interest of local media and weigh in with your perspective as health and mental health professionals.

CASE STUDY: REAUTHORIZATION OF THE SCHIP PROGRAM

The State Children's Health Insurance Program (SCHIP) was approved by Congress and the president in 1997. The program was designed to cover uninsured children in families with incomes that are modest but too high to qualify for Medicaid. It was expected to cover over six million children. The program, a partnership between the state and federal government, where states design their own programs according to the law, was approved and funded for 10 years through 2007, unless additional funds were subsequently appropriated.

Prior to the SCHIP deadline for reauthorization, children's advocacy groups began meeting with members of Congress to expand on the program. The group discussed which members of Congress were allies, certain or otherwise. They began to focus their efforts on those who were on the fence. Knowing that cost cutting was the focus of the members who did not support the program, the coalition shared with them data showing that routine care for children through this program reduced more expensive emergency room visits by the uninsured.

In 2007, the Democratic leadership of Congress proposed an expansion of SCHIP that would have extended federal health insurance coverage to an additional four million children in families, funded by a potential additional tax on cigarettes. H.R 967, Children's Health Insurance Program Reauthorization Act of 2007, was introduced in February and was sent to the House Ways and Means Committee for deliberation. The bill was drafted by the then-chair of the House Ways and Means Committee and, as a result, was fast tracked. The committee held hearings on the bill and its expansion. Partners of the coalition asked members of the committee to ask probing questions about the benefits of the program to the witnesses. Many child advocacy groups and coalitions were invited to provide testimony. The bill was then marked up with few amendments adopted. The House put the bill on calendar for debate the same day. The next day the chairman asked that the House suspend the rules and vote on the bill without amendments. There was a 40-minute debate on consideration of the suspension of the rules, then a vote in favor of suspending the rules, and then the bill was successfully passed. The bill was immediately sent to the Senate for consideration.

The Senate had not introduced its own bill and agreed to place the House bill on their calendar after its first reading. The Senate did not discuss the bill right away. Knowing that child advocacy groups were not the only ones in support of this bill, the coalition began to think about who could be additional allies—such as pediatric physician groups, education organizations, and labor unions. Now that they had a broader coalition, they began to meet in groups with legislators and their staffers to ensure that the Senate moved forward with the bill. Local town halls and rallies took place over the weekends and during recesses. The coalition knew that one of the major detractors of this bill was the tobacco industry, which was stating that the number of smokers was dwindling, so cigarette tax revenue would not provide enough funding for the expanded program. Television and newspaper ads, and letters to the editor from both sides of the argument, received attention in key congressional members' states and districts. These key members included Senate leadership and moderate Republican senators in states where the program was providing significant health care for kids. Five months after the bill was put on the Senate calendar, debate and amendments to the bill began. This lasted for 4 days when the Senate sent an amended version of the bill back to the House. The House eventually accepted the bill, which was sent to the president for signature. President Bush vetoed the legislation and the House was not successful by thirteen votes in overriding the veto—two-thirds vote is required.

Vowing not to let the program run out, Congress tried again to approve a similar bill, H.R. 3963, that would be more acceptable to the opposition. President Bush vetoed this legislation on December 12, 2007, and the House did not have a two-thirds majority to override.

As the deadline approached, many advocates knew a bill to continue the program needed to be adopted, or else millions of children would be left without insurance. In the end we knew we could build on the program at a later time but needed to ensure the program continued to run. On December 18, the Senate unanimously adopted S. 2499, to continue SCHIP funding until March 31, 2009, without the expansion. The House adopted the bill on December 19, and it was signed into law by President Bush on December 29, 2007.

For 2 years, child advocacy groups and coalitions worked with individual members of Congress to develop legislation to expand the program in 2009. On January 14, 2009, the House passed H.R. 2, Children's Health Insurance Program Reauthorization Act of 2009, on a vote of 290–138. The bill expanded the health coverage program to include about four million more children, including coverage of legal immigrants. A cigarette tax increase provided the additional funding for the program's expansion. On January 29, the Senate passed the House bill with two amendments. The House accepted the amended bill and President Obama signed the bill into law on February 4, 2009.

This case study shows how continuing relationships with elected officials, building on your coalition, and knowing your opposition is all essential. Also, knowing when to "get what you can" and not going down in flames is important. Although change could not happen in 2007, the program continued and further education prevailed 2 years later with the expansion of the program.

REFLECTION QUESTIONS

1. What different individuals or groups would support my cause? Who would oppose it?
2. What committees have jurisdiction over my issues of interest?
3. How can I make my elected official care about my cause?

PRACTICE MAKES PERFECT

1. Identify a bill currently before your state's legislature on a topic that you are interested in. What is the current status of the bill?
2. Track down the contact information for your U.S. Senators and House of Representatives. What e-mail address would you use to send them a short e-mail about an issue of importance to you?
3. Identify three organizations that could potentially be partners in advocacy on a specific issue of importance to you.

REFERENCES

Associated Press. (2008, April 26). *Wyoming senator Enzi announces reelection campaign, ending speculation.*
Domenici, P., & Wellstone, P. (2008). Mental Health Parity Act. Public Law No. 110–343.
Newport, F. (2009, August 12). Town hall meetings generate interest, some sympathy. *Gallup.*

5

How to Work With the Media

AARON LEVIN

I didn't have time to write a short letter, so I've written a long one instead.—Attributed to Mark Twain

Two sets of numbers impress policy makers: money and votes. The money we will leave to others, but convincing lawmakers that a significant number of voters in their districts care about and support a cause is an important part of advocacy.

Media extends advocacy's reach. Newspapers, radio, TV, websites, Facebook, Twitter, and their many variants can all amplify and repeat your message, reinforcing it in the minds of the public and legislators (Jerningan & Wright, 1996).

The more legislators believe that voters care about an issue, the more likely they are to act. Sometimes both voters and policy makers must first be shown that a problem exists and that someone (your advocacy group) has a solution. The media can bring an issue to widespread public attention, which can persuade policy makers about a desired course of action. How many constituents in the district will be affected if a policy is adopted or fails to pass? What will be the cost to the taxpayers? What are the substantive and political trade-offs between costs and benefits?

A media campaign is triangular. It works outward to the public to inform and spur them to discussion and action, and upward to legislators and regulators who hold the levers of power. Getting the public—or at least an interested segment—to inform the policy makers of their views completes the triangle (Figure 5.1).

Media exposure can be crucial in drawing the interest of an important intermediary group in the policy making process: the staff members who work for legislators. As mentioned in Chapter 4 on legislative

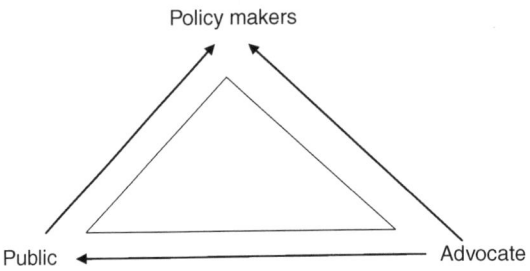

FIGURE 5.1
Directions of Influence in a Media Campaign

advocacy, influencing staffers is important, either by direct engagement or through the media. They are the gatekeepers for and interpreters of information about the district and the concerns of its citizens. They are publicly self-effacing, but their job is to understand both the issues and the politics of the issues and then present options and recommendations to the lawmaker.

Staff members at every level in legislative offices monitor news of the district or State, and track reports that mention the representative or Senator by name. Staffers also want to hear from advocacy groups. They know that medical professionals carry influence because they are regarded as experts, are credible, and are trusted by members of the community. Distance from the capital is no drawback because staffers for legislators monitor the websites of local news outlets to gauge local opinions. If a respected doctor or nurse appears on a local talk show or writes an op-ed article (so named because they are usually placed opposite the editorial page) appearing in a local paper, it will not go unnoticed. On some health issues, local experts can carry as much weight for their legislators as any Washington think tank.

THE MEDIA TODAY

"Media" is a plural noun and in an age of myriad streams of communication the plural has never been more appropriate. No one medium covers every audience. Once, everyone in town read the local newspaper every day and most Americans watched the network news in the evening. Not anymore. Many people, especially the youth, never read a daily newspaper, but they do have instant access to thousands of news sources that may originate anywhere on earth.

Desktop computers, laptops, tablets (iPads, Kindles, Nooks), iPods, smart cell phones, not-so-smart phones, palm tops, and more make up the new, always-changing digital universe. Each medium has its own charms and disadvantages, which the savvy advocate must consider.

Events can now appear in the media as they happen, in bits and chunks. Stories can be posted as soon as they are written. The time once taken to digest and distill the events a reporter covered may come only in the hours or days after a story breaks.

HOW DO I START?

As it is with most things in life, it is best to start at the end so you can figure out the best route from intention to objective. What do you want to achieve? What problem are you trying to solve? Are you trying to change regulations, expand the local hospital, construct a new research building, support or block proposed legislation, increase awareness of a threatening epidemic, or land a grant to expand care for the underserved?

How does this problem affect the community? (Community can mean your city, county, state, or the entire nation.) What solutions can you offer? Why are those solutions appropriate, relevant, cost-effective, or otherwise desirable? What competing (or opposing) proposals are part of the discussion? Why are yours better? Questions like these must be raised and answered before making any approach to the media, or before they come calling unannounced.

Each goal will determine its own path. Work backward to figure out what is needed to achieve success and what role media can play. Who needs to be persuaded? A governor? A legislative majority? Attentive members of the public? What will it take to persuade them? How best to achieve that end?

Planning the message takes more than the back of an envelope. Much of this background work probably took place at earlier stages in the advocacy process, when steering committees and task forces defined the problem and thrashed out the desired solution. The results of those discussions can be mined for ideas, words, and phrases to clarify your goal to the public.

Out of that material, begin by creating three versions of your message. First, boil the core message down to its simplest possible formulation, preferably a single—and not very long—sentence. State the problem, your solution, and the action needed. Next, develop a one-paragraph version—three or four sentences. Finally, craft a one-page version. You may want to have a more detailed and nuanced multi-paged case statement available to leave with policy makers or members of the media. A good reporter always wants as much raw material as possible.

At this point (and probably others, too), you may want to consult with the communications professionals in your organization or with public information officers in your hospital, university, or other institution.

CRAFTING THE MESSAGE

Pertaining to the quotation at the beginning of this chapter, when you plan a message, you want it to be like Goldilocks' porridge, not too long and not too short, but just right. In an age of e-mail, texting, and Twitter, attention spans grow shorter by the day. That does not mean that a long, discursive explanation of problems and solutions is entirely out of place, but it has to be targeted at an audience willing to read it. That is a key advantage of the digital realm. You can send a two-paragraph letter to the editor and link it to a 20-page, detailed case statement on your website.

EARNED MEDIA VERSUS PAID MEDIA

At this point, it may help to point out that what appears on news media is not all the same. Broadly speaking, what you see, hear, or read is divided into two parts. Call them news and advertising or, in media jargon, earned and paid media (Wallack & Dorfman, 2002). Earned media are what we think of as "content": news reports in any medium, op-eds, events or speeches, broadcast coverage, or interviews.

The subject of the story does not pay the media outlet to appear in earned media (or at least they are not supposed to). Decisions to report or run a story are made by editors and reporters who may or may not think your tale is worthy of coverage on any given day, compared to what else is going on in the neighborhood or the world.

Earned media is free in the sense that a sponsor does not pay for it, but gaining coverage does mean expending effort to understand the media's needs and preparing for appearances.

Reporters and editors need to fill time or space in order to attract audiences to the advertising that pays their bills. They are open to suggestion, but only if what you suggest fits their definition of content for their audience.

Paid media *is* advertising. Someone who wants to sell or promote something pays a fee to the outlet to buy time or space. Usually the boundary between earned and paid media is clearly marked.

Buying advertising takes up-front money, of course. Such funds come from an organization's treasury or through donations by members and supporters. No matter how large the advertising budget, however, the choice of media, the preparation of the ads, and the timing of their placement are under the control of the sponsor. Traditional media advertising is relatively simple compared to online advertising, but the latter offers some targeting options not available in newspapers or on radio and television. Online ads can be purchased to run next to search engine results or next to news stories relevant to your campaign's interests—on media websites.

However, the entire subject of the what, when, and where of advertising is a job for experienced specialists.

Finally, somewhere between paid and earned media lies the murky realm of audio and video news releases. In form, they appear to be news reports for radio or television with reporters holding microphones, but they are paid for by a sponsor, who is often not identified as such in the release. They are sent to radio and television stations, just as print news releases are sent out to news outlets. Like traditional press releases, they may be used as ideas for news stories by a local station, or they may simply be run as is, blending seamlessly into the station's regular newscast.

Many news outlets offer online chats, often with reporters or columnists. In format they are analogous to radio call-in shows, except that communication takes place by way of typed messages appearing on the viewer's screen. They have an advantage over radio in that guests have more time to compose their remarks and even edit them before hitting the "send" button. Participation still requires a well-prepared advocate.

GET TO KNOW YOUR MEDIA

Begin a media campaign by becoming familiar with the medium and who works for it. Understanding whom the outlet attracts as readers, viewers, or listeners is a key to knowing how to focus your message. For a peek behind the scenes at how the outlet views itself, ask for its media kit. This is the tool that media outlets use to inform and attract advertisers. It usually tells the number of readers, viewers, or listeners, where they live, how much they earn, how they divide up racially and ethnically, their marital status, and more. There may be clues as to their buying habits and their political views. Media kits are often online (here is one example: http://essentials.baltimoresun.com/media_kit/).

Another way to understand audiences is to read, view, or listen to the outlet. What is the content? How long are stories? How is the outlet structured? Are there lots of short pieces up front, followed by longer ones? What are the response mechanisms for readers, on- or offline? What can the mix of advertising tell you about readers?

How do you connect with people who work in the media? Reporters today all have e-mail addresses and blogs, Facebook pages, and Twitter accounts. All those categories now blur into one another. Your local newspaper not only lands on your doorstep in the morning, but it has been online all night on the paper's website, which may also include a video clip with an audio track and comments from readers. Who reads, watches, listens, follows friends, or tweets?

CONTACT LIST

Who covers health care or medicine or business for your local news outlets? Start by following their work. Who and what do they report about? Who do they quote as sources? Do they just rewrite press releases or can they get into the deeper meaning of a story? Just like police officers, journalists have "beats," in their case, subject areas they follow regularly. One reporter might have more than one beat. Depending on the issue for which you are advocating, you might aim your message at health, science, lifestyle, children's issues, or education reporters. Obviously, if one journalist has been reporting consistently on your topic, you should target that journalist. Since advocacy inevitably involves politics, reporters covering Congress or your State house when your issue arises should be included on your list, too.

A statewide list of media contacts might include dozens to hundreds of names of reporters and editors. A national list would contain thousands. E-mail is the preferred mode of communication today. (Although paper press releases are now so passe that they just might stand out from the crowd.) Sending e-mails is virtually free, but targeting your recipients is always a better approach.

Make the subject line pithy but interesting enough to move the recipient to click the "open" button and not "delete." A media release itself should be short—never more than the equivalent of one typed page—and should have an opening paragraph that contains the gist of the message. In some settings, particularly smaller markets, it may be possible to meet face-to-face with a reporter before stories arise. This represents an opportunity to establish your credentials as a source and as an advocate well before the reporter is on a deadline. Be aware that any conversation with a reporter, however informal it seems at the time, is fair game for inclusion in an article or column unless you place it off the record in advance.

When major issues arise, the editorial board of a news outlet may want to talk to advocates in order to inform an editorial. To connect with a reporter, try an e-mail as a first approach. Individualize your message. "Dear Susan," works better than "Dear Reporter." Follow up with a phone call a day or two later. They may or may not have seen your e-mail. Make your introduction brief and your pitch concise: "I am the vice-president of the state nurses association and I would like to talk to you about the patient safety implications of proposed hospital staffing requirements in the health care bill now before the House of Delegates."

Answers are likely to be "Yes," "No," or "Not now." Leave your name and contact information. You may be asked to follow up with another e-mail. Do so immediately. Keep in mind, too, that the entire news business is in deep flux now. Major organizations have laid off staff and the remaining personnel must produce more in less time than ever before.

It still may be possible to take a reporter to lunch, but do not bet on it. Establish yourself as a local expert. Having letters such as MD, RN, MSW, DDS, and PharmD after your name is a good start. So are other credentials that indicate your expertise, such as being an officer in your local or national professional association or holding a faculty position at a university. However, this is not the time to attach your complete curriculum vitae (CV). In fact, there is rarely a time to attach your complete CV. Define your role, especially as it applies to the topic of at hand: a pediatric dentist, a geriatric nurse, a health care economist, a preventive medicine specialist, and so on. This should tie in the cause and current action. It is unlikely that a reporter will be interested in your expertise unless there is a story to go with it. Use upcoming local events—rallies, health screening days—as news pegs, also called hooks, but remember to pitch your ideas well in advance of the outlet's deadlines.

Contacts with reporters and editors can be important down the road. Do not pepper them with trivia, but when you have a good story idea, or it is crunch time for your campaign in the legislature, a personal e-mail or call may reap coverage. And when that reporter leaves you a message saying she wants to talk to you about your campaign (or anything else), please call back as soon as possible. Deadlines are deadlines and if she does not hear from you in time, she will surely track down someone else, who may or may not agree with you.

A small-market newspaper or broadcast station may be receptive to a periodic column or call-in program. However, you must be a good writer and meet deadlines unfailingly for that to work. Such projects serve better to establish your visibility and credibility than pushing your advocacy position. A column creates recognition that can improve your status as an expert when the need for advocacy arises.

PREPARING FOR INTERVIEWS

Interviews are an important part of any media campaign. Again, prepare by watching, listening, or reading the medium or outlet. Get a sense of how interviews flow. Will you be interviewed for the top-of-the-hour news cast that might extract a single, short sentence, or will you sit on an hour-long call-in show? Is the interviewer neutral and polite, deferential and flattering, or aggressive and possibly even hostile? Sometimes it is hard to know in advance.

Write down your talking points before the interview, including your personal stories. Data may not be the plural of anecdote, but a good story never hurts provided it is short and to the point. "I remember when I was in medical school and a little child died because of the lack of [whatever]. We want to be sure that no child ever has to go through that again. That's why this bill has to pass." Always consider opposing points of view and prepare answers to counter those points because they will very likely be raised during your interview.

Interviews are like playing the piano. The more you practice, the better you get. Ask a colleague or family member to quiz you beforehand. Try to anticipate likely questions and prepare answers. Or try saying your keys lines into a recorder and listening to what you sound like. Practice until it sounds more natural.

INTERVIEW BASICS

Begin by stating your message and stating it early. One media specialist says that no matter how long the interview is scheduled to last, get your main point out in the first 30 seconds. Use questions as springboards to reiterate your message. Experts call this "pivoting": "That's true, Bob, but with more research money we could make a real dent in the problem."

AVOID JARGON AND ACRONYMS

Your working life may abound with TLAs (three-letter acronyms) but they will leave a lay audience (and most legislators) puzzled or even angry. Inside language looks like snobbishness to outside audiences. Plain language that uses English rather than polysyllabic Latin always carries more force, anyway: "Heart attack" sounds much punchier than "myocardial infarction," right?

Never get defensive or argumentative, and try to avoid the "off the record" statements. If you do not want some casual remark to come back and bite you, do not say it. Also, "I don't know" is a perfectly acceptable answer, especially when you do not know the answer. Do not fake it. If you are not sure of a statistic or your organization's position on something, say, "I will get back to you on that." Then check with your leadership or the relevant authority and call the reporter back as soon as possible. Do the same if you realize afterward that you misstated some point. It may be possible to correct it before airtime.

Remember, assume that all microphones are live. Many a politician has lived to regret an inapt remark that was unknowingly recorded or broadcast.

Be concise. The way to be concise is to plan ahead. Boil your arguments down to talking points. Then boil those down to a single sentence. The ideal quote in any medium is not a detailed recital of facts but a pithy illumination of an otherwise confusing landscape.

Finally, articulate your campaign's message in your own words but be consistent with colleagues. Offering your own personal views (when they differ from the campaign's) when you are acting as an official spokesperson gives opponents or the media a chance to point out and exploit inconsistencies.

INTERVIEWS AND TELEVISION

Media training for television is an art in itself. Much can be learned from an online search on the phrase, but anyone who frequently represents an organization or a cause on television or radio should avail him- or herself of formal media training by an expert. More than one person in an organization should have the training to undertake media interviews.

Try to get a video recording of your segment (or have someone at home record it). Analyze your performance—and yes, it is a "performance"—to better understand your deficiencies and your strengths. Get advice, or figure out what you did well, how well your message came across, and what can be improved (Chapman, 2004; Hearne, 2008). Send the clip to your legislator. If the segment will be aired in the future, let your legislator's office know when your story will be run.

Follow every media contact with an e-mail thanking the reporter for the opportunity to chat and reminding her about your availability for further questions. You may get calls or re-mails after an interview seeking answers for follow-up questions. Those questions come late in the production process, when the clock is ticking toward press time or airtime, so respond as soon as possible.

LETTERS TO THE EDITOR

Once this meant actual letters to newspapers, but many of the same principles can be applied to comments sections of websites or blogs. Today, nearly all letters to the editor are sent by e-mail or through forms on the outlet's website. Many reporters will print or post incoming missives sent via Twitter, Facebook, or cell phone text.

Letters to the editor usually are responses to published stories or prior letters or to some recent event. They can also be used to spark public awareness at crucial moments, such as just before the legislature is getting ready to vote on your topic. Reply to daily papers or websites quickly, ideally within 24 hours. Weekly newspapers have longer deadlines.

If letters are in response to published comments by your campaign's opponents, summarize their point(s) very succinctly, in one sentence or less, then move on to counter those points and make your own points positively. Name-calling or mud-slinging are neither good manners nor good strategy. Brevity is best. Many outlets have word limits. Find out in advance what they are and do not exceed them. Web comment forms often have built-in limits. Your message, no matter how diligently you slaved over it, may simply be discarded if it is too long. And editing your own letter for length means that you, not the editor, get to keep what is most important in your message. Cover only one main point, not a laundry list of issues or minor points.

Always include full contact information, including office address, phone, and e-mail address. Outlets use these to verify the writer's identity. Again, be sure to tack on your qualifying higher degrees after your name (MD, RN, PhD). Some papers limit the number of letters in a given month or year from a single writer. Ask about that. If you need to send letters more frequently, consider having other members of your advocacy group send them in their names. Generally, do not list more than two signers, even if the letter comes from a group.

If your campaign is centrally coordinated, run your letter past the communications staff person or other media coordinator, if possible. They will give you good suggestions for keeping on message and maintaining the proper tone. Better yet, consult with them early on before you start to write. Do not cut and paste form letters prepared by your organization and e-mailed to all members. Editors will immediately recognize them as canned responses and are less likely to publish them. Better to have one person carefully craft a single original letter than to have 50 form letters with the same wording arrive on an editor's desk. Petitions may work to impress Congresspeople but content rather than numbers are more likely to get published in traditional news media. And always, always proofread the letter. Then get someone else to proofread it.

Understand the comments policies of websites. Some permit anything to appear in the comments to articles online. Others are moderated, meaning that an actual human being reviews comments, usually for name-calling or other nasty language but often for content. Comment periods are often limited. Be selective in responding. Too often, comments are mere rants, so a brief, well-crafted response stands out.

OP-EDS

Newspaper op-eds still have a special place in the world of communications, even in the day of the 140-character Tweet and the 15-second attention span.

An op-ed is an opinion piece, usually written by a person not on the paper's editorial board. Often, the opinions expressed are buttressed by facts, although the facts are selected by the writer. An artfully written op-ed dropped before the public's eye at the right time can still serve to initiate or advance a cause. Op-eds may inform legislative thinking and even language. Print is still the benchmark of journalism, no matter how much it seems to be the poor cousin at the media party. Opportunities for longer form discussions exist all over the web, too, but the discipline imposed by the op-ed form can keep a writer from rambling and an audience engaged.

First, obtain guidelines for the op-ed. Often, these are posted on the outlet's website. If not, call or e-mail to find out. For example, one paper's website says it "welcomes submissions of op-ed articles of 650 to 750 words. Local topics and authors are preferred." Take those standards seriously. The editor responsible for the op-ed page does not have the time to edit your 1,000-word op-ed down to 750 words. Local authorship, on the other hand, represents an opportunity. Write for your local paper and you are not in competition with the people who write op-eds in the *New York Times* or *Washington Post*. The op-ed should present a point of view, but one that is supported with data and good reasoning.

Ask a colleague and your communications team to read over your op-ed for both style and content before you send it. Follow these pointers:

- Be accurate and on message.
- Be timely. Link your op-ed to a recent news event that shows how your cause can help people in the community. Or tie it to some, even slightly, newsworthy aspect of your campaign—a rally, a health screening, or appearance by a local celebrity, for instance.
- Be local. Refer only passingly to any national aspects of the campaign and be sure to show the local need and benefits of the cause.

Once the op-ed is published, post it on your campaign website and send out notes on Twitter or by e-mail to draw readers to it. If it does not get picked up at first, submit it elsewhere. Op-eds raise the profile not only of the issue, but of the writer. For a time, at least, the op-ed writer becomes the local authority on the issue and a de facto leader.

MEDIA OPPORTUNITIES

Press conferences, briefings, and media events are important adjuncts to a campaign. Schedule them for early in the day, so reporters can meet deadlines for evening newscasts and the following morning's newspapers. Press conferences usually consist of one or a few individuals making brief statements to the press and taking follow-up questions from reporters.

Briefings may involve more detailed presentations of research material or other background material. Often, speakers may include not just experts but also individuals affected by the issue, adding a personal and anecdotal layer to the information. These personal tales frequently lead off news coverage, which then go into the less-accessible but more significant aspects of related policy. Consider holding press briefings with coalition partners. The combination not only draws more attention but helps lessen claims that the proposed policy is just a turf battle or a matter of money.

Both types of events can be organized as in-person events, attended by reporters, or as virtual events or webinars complete with audio, slides, and video, and the ability to take phoned-in or e-mailed questions. Such technologies can expand the event's reach when reporters cannot attend in person because of time or distance constraints.

Media events generally involve a bit of theatricals. They are designed to create visuals for the benefit of cameras. The drama draws media attention, as when doctors picket a theater to protest positive depictions of smoking.

SHARE YOUR SUCCESS

Learn from your mistakes and keep refining your message. Encourage colleagues to make time to work with media. Keep going!

THE DIGITAL REALM

An online presence is essential for any advocacy campaign. For one thing, a website is the norm by now. If your views are not represented on the web, they will be lost to sight. There are other advantages, too. A news story, however favorable, is a distillation of the reporter's newsgathering and usually abbreviated for time or space. A website allows the unaltered presentation of your point of view.

Spend the time and money for an expert to design your website. Standards are now high. Viewers form instant impressions about organizations from their websites' appearance and navigation qualities. Do not forget that websites need constant updating, too.

SOCIAL MEDIA

Social media are required tracks as well, especially for younger members. Websites now include links to social media sites like Facebook and Twitter or social news sharing sites like Digg and Reddit. All of these require care and feeding, and it may be necessary to hire or assign someone to keep them updated.

Activity on social media cannot stand alone. It must flow organically from every other aspect of the advocacy campaign. Social media should not be viewed as simply another information channel. Their interactivity is the essence of their nature, not merely another handy feature. In the minds of their participants, the purpose of social media is to develop a transparent community (or something that looks like it). To build that affinity, the host of the page must gain the trust of participants and be open to their interaction.

Thus, pages on Facebook must be frequently updated and a monitor must respond to comments. The ethos there includes a call to action: "Read this. Check this out. Write to your Congressman. DO something!" Facebook provides its subscribers with counts of numbers of visitors, along with some of the demographic data required from members at sign-up. This information can be helpful in understanding who is interested in or responding to your campaign. Twitter, with its 140-character-per-Tweet limit, is probably not the best way to explain a complex, nuanced piece of legislation that involves law, science, and finance. However, it can be used as an alert system to get members of an organization to act or respond to some event. For instance, if a bill is about to be voted on in the State legislature, organization members can be alerted to call or e-mail their representatives (with the bill number included) to express their views. Alternatively, they can be directed to the organization's website to read a fuller explanation.

Twitter can be used to send information to constituents but it may be even more valuable for tracking the public's current interests, seeding ideas into ongoing discussions, and feeding items to the news media.

One may fantasize about having a video clip go viral on YouTube or other social video sites but as often as not, it is likely to happen for the wrong reasons. The video clips that get airplay on YouTube seem to be (a) funny; (b) embarrassing; or (c) on pop culture. However, posting a well-produced short segment that demonstrates the problem you are trying to solve and then presents your position can both engage an audience and link them to your other web or online points.

Specialized blogs serve the role that specialized newsletters once did, but with some added informality. Blogs can aggregate and link to lots of other information sources. The most successful blogs include frequent updates to bring viewers back repeatedly. Once again, that argues for assigning someone to write frequently—as often as once a day, or at least every few days. The updates can be brief and can link to news reports or other sites of interest.

Social media are still evolving. They have the power to assist a campaign, but also to cause harm and create backlashes. For that reason, planning the entire communications process and coordinating its elements are essential. The impulsive, spontaneous nature of internet communications may not always be a campaign's best friend. Anything that goes out on the web should be considered "published" in the fullest sense of "made public," so advocates must take care to reach their intended audience with carefully chosen words and images. Timing is also important. You don't want a legislator's staffer making up her/his mind before you talk to her/him and explain your views.

FINAL THOUGHTS

The more organized and coordinated an advocacy media campaign, the better. Advanced planning, maintaining a consistent core message through all media, and integrating that effort with direct lobbying provide the greatest likelihood of success. Advocates must follow up, repeat their message, energize the public, and move them to action to convince policy makers to make the desired choices.

In many cases, advocacy organizations may do well to hire a media relations professional to plan and carry out many of the activities discussed here. Nevertheless, any advocate can benefit by understanding the processes outlined above.

CASE STUDY: HEALTHY MINDS, HEALTHY LIVES

In 2005, the American Psychiatric Association (APA) began its "Healthy Minds, Healthy Lives" campaign with two goals in mind: to change the way the public thought about psychiatry and psychiatrists, and to reduce the stigma associated with mental illnesses. The campaign was designed and managed by the APA's Office of Communications and Public Affairs and the public relations firm of Porter Novelli.

The campaign's target audience was women aged 30 to 54, who were seen as "health gatekeepers for their families and open to seeing a mental health professional." The organization used focus groups and surveys to plan the campaign, which linked psychiatry and psychiatrists (all of whom are medical doctors) to overall health.

The APA enlisted five spokespersons: three high ranking officers (all women) of the organization, including the President-Elect; the mother of a child with attention deficit hyperactivity disorder; and the (male) Director of the APA's research division. All had received or were given media training for the campaign.

The APA and Porter Novelli developed media training materials and talking points for the spokespersons: brochures and fact sheets, website contents, and media kits with news releases, survey results, and spokesperson biographies. The website drew nearly one million visitors in its first year (May 2005 to May 2006).

Two strategies were used to increase viewership. The APA purchased advertising on the popular search engine sites Google and Yahoo. They also focused mini-campaigns within the main project on college mental health, Hispanic audiences (with Spanish translations of fact sheets and other materials), and Mental Health Awareness Week.

The campaign sent out an audio news release to 600 radio stations and arranged for a satellite media tour, in which spokespersons based in a studio in Washington, DC, can hold interviews with television and radio reporters around the country. The APA estimated that these efforts reached a potential audience of 105 million broadcasts listeners and viewers and four million readers of print or online media.

REFLECTION QUESTIONS

1. How can a media campaign be best timed to exert influence on policy makers during the legislative or regulatory process?
2. Pick an advocacy cause dear to you. How can social media be integrated into your advocacy efforts?
3. Discuss ways to pare a statement about your campaign—word-by-word, if necessary—down to its essence.

PRACTICE MAKES PERFECT

1. Write a two-paragraph letter to the editor, in less than 100 words, about a cause for which you wish to advocate.
2. Write four talking points you would use for an interview with a reporter about this cause—no more than one sentence each.
3. Come up with a memorable domain name (e.g., www.mywebsite.org) for your cause. Make sure the domain name has not been claimed already, and investigate online for possible web designers to build this website for you.

REFERENCES

Chapman, S. (2004). Advocacy for public health: A primer. *Journal of Epidemiology & Community Health Health*, 58(5), 361–365.

Hearne, S. A. (2008). Practice-based teaching for health policy action and advocacy. *Public Health Reports, 123*(Suppl. 2), 65–70.
Jerningan, D. H., & Wright, P. (1996). Media advocacy: Lessons from community experiences. *Journal of Public Health Policy, 17*(3), 306–330.
Wallack, L., & Dorfman, L. (2002). Putting policy into health communication: The role of media advocacy. In R. E. Rice & C. K. Atkin (Eds.), *Public Communication Campaigns* (3rd ed., pp. 389–401). Thousand Oaks, CA: Sage.

6

Is There a Lawyer in the House? When to Work With an Attorney

SARAH S. WESSELS AND MEGAN SANDEL

Far more has been accomplished for the welfare and progress of mankind by preventing bad actions than by doing good ones.—William Lyon Mackenzie King

Health care providers use their medical training to help patients solve health issues every day. Beyond the hospital or clinic environment, a patient may face challenges that compromise the care provided by medical expertise alone, and may even seriously affect their overall quality of life. Some less fortunate patients become highly indebted due to the costs of their care. Other patients may go home to an environment that poses significant health risks. These are examples where patients' unmet legal needs may complicate their health condition, and legal solutions may be essential parts of effective care.

An *unmet legal need* is a situation in which *the patient does not recognize that a problem has a legal solution*. These legal solutions are often unknown to patients because they are misguided by a *legal myth, a common misunderstanding about legal rights*, which prevents them from seeking legal help. The types of legal needs that are discussed in this chapter often cause embarrassment, pose risks to patients' personal well-being, or both. As a result, patients may avoid discussing their situations with peers or government agencies. This means that as a health care provider, you may be in a special position of confidence, a unique position as the only informed persons aware of a *patient's private circumstances*. In this position, you may be the only person who can correct the misunderstanding and empower the patient to connect with a *potential legal solution*.

Legal advocacy can initially be as simple as suggesting a patient consider legal help. As your sophistication in this advocacy evolves, you may start to develop expanded intake forms, provide informative handouts in the office, and create your own medical–legal partnership (MLP).

In this chapter, we cover key principles of case-based advocacy, meaning advocacy work on behalf of individual cases. See Chapter 7 to learn more about collaboration with attorneys on behalf of large groups of patients and class action lawsuits. Here we review the following:

1. **Unmet legal needs:** By surveying the most common unmet legal needs, we will show their health connections ("health-ties"), reveal their underlying legal myths, show examples of common situations in which these occur, and provide tips on how to connect affected patients with the best potential legal solutions.
2. **How to refer a patient** to the right legal resources for their circumstance.
3. **Medical–legal partnership:** As patient support services develop and become an official component of patient care, they are able to provide a more sophisticated network of resources for both health care professionals and the patients themselves.
4. **Advocating for policy changes:** Sometimes patients' issues go beyond just their own medical and legal needs. Health care professionals periodically encounter important opportunities to improve the guiding policies impacting effective care. We will conclude this section with some resources for tackling policy change.

IDENTIFYING UNMET LEGAL NEEDS

A tool that can be useful in remembering common unmet legal needs is the acronym **IHELP**:

I: Insurance and Income: making sure patients have food, cash, and do not ignore health problems for insurance reasons
H: Housing: finding and staying in a safe and clean home
E: Education and Employment: adjusting education and employment to accommodate health conditions
L: Legal Status: accessing rights and overcoming concerns about deportation
P: Personal and Family Security: preventing domestic violence and creating plans for incapacity and death

Unmet Legal Need I: Income

Health-tie. Without income, a patient may decide to forego basic life necessities (food, water, and a place to stay).

Legal myth. Many patients believe that their sole source of income and insurance is their employer. This is not true. Everyone in this country can potentially qualify for other sources of income and insurance (see Table 6.1) and *we do not have to deplete our assets to zero* before we access these benefits.

Each of these agencies has a website that includes relevant criteria, necessary forms, and an overview of the application process. For the Social Security Administration visit www.ssa.gov, and for all other types

TABLE 6.1
Income as a Solution

Patient Circumstance	Type of Benefit	Where to Go to Apply
Cannot work because of an injury or illness (short-term)	Private disability insurance	Insurance provider or state economic development agency
	Worker's compensation[1]	
Permanently disabled (cannot work for one year or more)	Private disability insurance	Insurance provider
	Social security disability income[2]	Social security administration
	Supplemental security income[3]	Supplemental security administration
Laid-off from job	Unemployment income[4]	State economic development agency
Cares for children or ill family member	Public need-based benefits such as temporary assistance for needy families (commonly known as welfare)[5]	County welfare office
Recently divorced or care for young children	Child support and spousal support[6]	Department of child support services
		Family law court
Recently lost spouse or is a disabled child who lost supporting parent	Social security survivors benefits[7]	Social security administration
	Veterans benefits[8]	Department of Veteran Affairs
Does not fit in other category	General assistance[9]	County welfare department
	Supplemental nutritional access program (SNAP)[10]	Utility provider
	Utility costs reduction programs[11]	

of benefits, the patient can search the Internet for "[type of benefit] in [patient's state]" and he or she should be able to find the nearest office. In many counties patients can dial 211 for information on public benefits.

Tips for income issues. Most of these public benefit options have a rather straightforward application process. An attorney is useful for patients who have been denied benefits, or for those who would like to have a confidential discussion about their personal circumstances, such as how their immigration status may affect income.

Tips for utility issues. Low-income populations may be eligible for discounted utilities or for Low Income Home Energy Assistance Program (LIHEAP) dollars that can prevent patients from falling behind on bills. Lastly, legal services can help families put together payment plans or automatic draws on public benefits that can pay down utility debt and avoid shut-offs.

CASE STUDY: FOOD AND UTILITIES[12]

J.S., age 58, was diagnosed with advanced head and neck cancer. He and his wife live 2 hours from the cancer center and receive food stamps. Rather than drive back and forth each day for his radiation treatments, he elected to stay at a local hospitality room. The Division of Social Services learned that he was not residing in his home and reduced their food stamp benefits by more than half. In addition, he and his wife needed immediate heating assistance because the gas company threatened to turn off their heat for failure to pay their bills.

A legal services attorney was able to schedule an immediate fair hearing for his food stamp reduction, increasing the benefits above the previous rate. The attorney was also able to obtain emergency assistance from the Home Energy Assistance Program (HEAP) for his heating. By resolving these two immediate concerns, the patient was able to remain in the hospitality house to complete his radiation therapy before returning home.

Unmet Legal Need I: Insurance

Health-tie. Without insurance, treatable health conditions may become life-threatening emergencies.

Legal myth. "We do not have public health insurance in this country."

Potential legal solutions; insurance. A patient may be entitled to the following:

- Federally funded programs such as Medicare and Medicaid[13] for the young and disabled, or veterans' health benefits
- Private health insurance extensions under the Consolidated Omnibus Budget Reconciliation Act (COBRA)[14]; they may be able to appeal an improper cancelation of private insurance
- State and local health programs[15] that provide insurance coverage for specific issues such as pregnancy, cancer screening, and sexual disease testing, sometimes regardless of immigration status

Tips for insurance issues. State programs provide a wide variety of insurance options to help young adults with limited income. For families with serious health conditions that have some assets, such as a home, a lawyer can help the family plan for need-based insurance and other types of public benefits. For example, a patient can receive Medicaid (public health insurance for financially needy individuals) and keep his home and the tools required for his work, and use the resulting savings to pre-pay property taxes and utility bills.[16] Furthermore, for a married patient, her spouse is entitled to keep her share of savings and investments.[17]

Unmet Legal Need H: Housing (Access to Housing and Utilities, Availability, and Allergens)

Health-tie. A critical step in any patient's recovery is a safe place to stay. Vulnerable populations may *face eviction*, have difficulty *accessing a home*, or have problems related to the quality and upkeep of their rental unit (*habitability*.) Without access to this critical resource, patients may find themselves with expensive and/or frequent emergency room visits with serious but preventable health conditions.

Legal myths:

Homeowners: *"If I miss a mortgage or rent payment, I can always be legally evicted."*
Renters: *"Housing provided by 'Section 8' is for the extremely poor and the apartments are not safe."*

Potential legal solutions:

- *Eviction from rental units.* If patients are being evicted for not paying rent, they may have a defense if they are disabled and the problem can be remedied with a *reasonable accommodation*[18] (an adjustment to the terms of the lease to make it more fair to the disabled tenant), if there were habitability problems[19] (the unit was not clean or safe), or if the landlord unlawfully raised the rent in violation of a rent-control ordinance. Some cities have nonprofit organizations that will help needy families make a one-time rent payment.

- *Foreclosure defense.* The patient may have rights under the Making Homes Affordable Act[20] to *decrease the amount of their mortgage payment* during treatment for a serious health condition.
- *Rental access.* Federal housing assistance is based on the median income for the area. Many families with mid-range income may still qualify. While public housing developments are one option, there are also government voucher programs, known as "Section 8" vouchers, that can help cover the rent in an existing rental unit in which the individual feels comfortable and safe.[21]

Tips for eviction issues. Evicting a tenant is often an expensive option for a landlord. If the tenant is represented, the attorney can help him or her identify wrongdoing or negotiate a settlement that is better for both parties. These agreements may include provisions in which the tenant has an opportunity to catch up on rent over several months. The best-case scenario from the tenant's perspective is when an attorney can find an *illegal rent increase*, and the landlord owes the tenant back-payment of rent.

For homeowners, a lawyer can review the terms of the mortgage for *illegal financing terms*[22] and may be able to slow down or prevent the foreclosure. Sometimes there are purchase options available with banks that will not affect the homeowner's credit, such as a *deed in lieu of foreclosure.*[23]

CASE STUDY: EVICTION DEFENSE[24]

J.D., age 43, was diagnosed with terminal cervical cancer and admitted into a hospital for pain management. She was a single mother of two teenage children. After hospitalization she fell behind on rent and soon thereafter received an eviction notice in her federally subsidized home.

J.D.'s case was referred to a local legal services program attorney who inspected the apartment and found the landlord had not kept the apartment in a livable condition. The attorney presented this information to the housing board, and the board found that the landlord was also at fault. Instead of being evicted and having to find a new unsubsidized apartment, J.D. was moved by the housing board into the next available unit. If not for the legal intervention, she would have been evicted, and the children of a very sick, homeless mother would have been placed in foster care. The patient was able to spend 2 weeks at home with her children prior to her death. After she died, the attorney assisted the patient's grandmother with gaining custody of the two children.

Legal myth. "Part of living in a city (or low-income housing) is living with mice, mold, and cockroaches; these pests are inconvenient, but not dangerous."

Potential legal solutions for habitability issues. Asthma and allergies can be significantly affected by poor building maintenance, therefore every lease has an implied *warranty of habitability*, which means that the landlord must remove pests at their expense regardless of how much the tenant pays or where the unit is located. Depending on state law, tenants may be entitled to self-help remedies such as a *reduction in rent*, the right to *fix the problem and deduct the cost from rent*, or to *abandon their lease* in favor of an inhabitable environment to help cover the costs of fixing the problems themselves.[25]

Tips for allergen issues. Encouragement from a doctor that eye infections, skin rashes, asthma and allergies are serious health risks that can be critical in getting a patient to connect their housing to their health. If health care providers are willing to send a letter recording the severity of the problem, this can be useful in getting a landlord to act.

CASE STUDY: MICE ARE THREATS TO HEALTH[26]

Three-year-old Jessica kept getting sick. In one winter alone, she was taken to the emergency room three times for pneumonia, and she was losing weight and developing rashes. Candice, Jessica's mother, thought the mice in her apartment were making her daughter sick. She asked her building manager repeatedly to exterminate the mice, but the answer was always the same: There was no money for it. Besides, the building manager said, a company was already coming every 3 months to set traps.

Candice found help at the local MLP for children (MLPC), where she met with the directing attorney. After receiving a letter and a couple of phone calls detailing the building manager's legal responsibility to keep the unit clean, the building manger hired a new, better-equipped exterminator to deal with the infestation. The program worked and Jessica no longer suffers from pneumonia or rashes.

Unmet Legal Need E: Education

Health-tie. Regardless of whether the health problem comes in the form of an acute health crisis or a chronic condition, a child's health is going to affect his academic performance.

Legal myth. "Teachers are in the best position to identify a child's needs and to recommend a course of action."

Potential legal solutions for education issues. Children have the following rights:

- Attend school regardless of their *legal status* and *parents' financial status*
- Attend the same school they went to before they became *homeless* or moved to a more convenient location
- Receive school meals, special education, and transportation, and cannot be denied enrollment because they cannot find or access requested documents (immunization records, birth certificates, etc.)[27]
- Be tested for learning disabilities and receive special education for diagnosed disabilities[28]
- Request changes to the learning environment to make it easier for them to succeed if they have a health condition that affects their education[29]

Potential legal solutions for special needs. While teachers are a critical piece of success, the best advocacy is going to involve a team approach. Parents have a right to request a *special needs assessment* and an *individual education plan* to help children with special needs succeed.

Tips for special needs issues. It costs the school time and money to address special needs. If the child goes to a school that is tight on finances, the parents may need to adamantly pursue action to get results. The parent may consider contacting an education attorney who can appeal a decision by the school board. Furthermore, education attorneys are often connected to community resources that can help parents identify the type of support they want the school to provide.

CASE STUDY: SPECIAL NEEDS FOR CHILD WITH CEREBRAL PALSY[30]

Jane is a devoted mother trying to make the best life possible for her children. Her 11-year-old, hearing-impaired daughter named Grace has cerebral palsy. Jane told Grace's pediatrician she was concerned her daughter's struggles in school were due to a lack of special support. The pediatrician referred Jane to Children's Law Center (CLC) to help Grace get the equipment and resources she needed for her special health and education challenges.

The CLC attorney, Yael, worked as a fierce advocate to ensure Grace received the support she needed to thrive in school. Thanks to Yael's persistence and dedication to her client, Grace can now easily complete her homework with an at-home tutor in a desk that enables her to read and write with no limitations. She keeps up in school and no longer falls behind her peers.

Legal myth. "School punishment is necessary for children with behavioral issues."

Potential legal solution for health-related behavioral problems. If a child has a serious health condition affecting their behavior, the school must discuss what types of reasonable accommodations, or changes to the learning environment, will help the child. Discipline alone is not always acceptable.

Tips for behavioral problem issues. A lawyer working with the child's doctor can help identify the source of the problems and request the school to make changes to the classroom rules to accommodate the health needs of the child. For instance, a child with hearing problems may get bored when she cannot understand the teacher, and then cause class disruptions. Working with the parents and teachers, lawyers can often negotiate a solution that does not require punishment, such as moving the student to the front of the class or to a classroom with better acoustics.

Unmet Legal Need E: Employment

Health-tie. Health conditions affect an entire family's ability to prosper. Frequent absences or tardiness, inability to focus and complete tasks on time, and poor teamwork are often tied to the side effects of medication, an ill family member, or chronic pain.

Legal myth. "If an employee runs out of sick leave or is too sick to perform his job duties, the employer can lay him off."

Potential legal solutions for employment issues. A patient has the following rights:

- Ask for time off to treat a medical condition, such as rights under the Federal Family Medical Leave Act (FMLA)[31]
- Request changes to the work environment or schedule to accommodate a condition including schedule changes or position changes[32]
- Negotiate job and benefits protection during a period of absence to treat a medical condition[33]

Family members taking care of a seriously ill relative should be aware of two rights:

- The right to take time off to care for a seriously ill family member with job protection and benefits protection under the Family Medical Leave Act[34]

- Some states provide paid time off for employees caring for a seriously ill family member such as the California Paid Leave Act[35]

Tips for employment issues. While there are many protections for ill employees, *patients must communicate their health problems to their employer* to be protected. Employees often miss out on important protections because they do not want their employer to know they are ill, or want to keep the nature of their condition private.

The employee does not have to discuss the specifics of her disease; she just has to let her employer know she has a health condition that is affecting her work. Once on notice, the employer has a legal duty to at least discuss changes to work conditions that can accommodate the needs of the employee. Examples of reasonable accommodations include requesting a later start time for pregnant women with morning sickness, or shifting from the sales floor to the office for an elderly patient healing from a hip fracture. In taking time off for treatment and recovery, many job losses are due to failing to keep in touch with an employer or a benefit company. Asking for legal help or requesting that a caregiver be contacted in addition to the patient can help prevent missed communications.

CASE STUDY: DISABILITY BENEFIT DENIALS[36]

John, a 53-year-old executive, was used to living on a six-figure income, navigating the complex demands of his work, home life, and finances. One afternoon during a routine staff meeting, John found that he was too confused to finish his presentation. His doctor found that John's symptoms were caused by the HIV virus and immediately put him on medication that could prolong his life. The medication interfered with his mental clarity and John soon found he could no longer work. He left work on a short-term disability program. A few months later, his benefits payments stopped. When he called the insurance company, they told him they were ending his benefits because the problem was a preexisting condition and not covered under the policy. Furthermore, they claimed to have sent him notice and the period for contesting the decision had passed.

That is when Susan, a local disability rights attorney and AIDS Legal Referral Panel (ALRP) member, stepped in. As John's cash was running low, Susan agreed to take the case on a *contingency basis* and immediately filed suit. After sending the insurance company a strongly worded memo summarizing recent court decisions, they settled the suit promptly. Although John was not able to go back to work, he was able to stay in his home and live his life with dignity and respect.

Unmet Legal Need L: Legal Status

Health-tie. Patients may decide to forego seeking necessary health benefits because of fear of deportation. A lawyer can help these patients understand what public benefits are available and if there are risks involved in applying.

Legal myth. "State or federal government agencies will report undocumented immigrants if they apply for benefits."

Potential legal solutions:
- Food stamp offices may not deny an application for food stamps because one member of a household is not eligible.[37]
- Children can usually get benefits such as food stamps regardless of the parent's legal status.
- Undocumented immigrants may qualify for Social Security Administration benefits such as Medicare and retirement or disability income if they have significant U.S. work history.[38]
- Parents can seek child support and spousal support from another parent working in this country (legally or illegally).
- Immigrants can always go to a hospital to receive necessary health care and immunizations for children.[39]
- Refugees who flee a country in fear of their lives or the lives of their children may be entitled to become citizens for humanitarian reasons.[40] U-VISAs, discussed below, may be available for crime victims.[41]

Tips for legal status issues. If you have a patient who fled in fear of his or her life or safety, offering to sign a *declaration in support* can be critical to immigration hearings. Judges tend to dismiss claims of abuse unless a doctor has evaluated the client and signed a declaration showing signs of abuse. Local legal services programs are a good resource for finding a lawyer who can help the family members identify what public benefits are available in their state and what the state's procedures are for requesting information about the parents.

Unmet Legal Need P: Personal and Family Stability

Health-tie. More than any other community group, health care professionals often identify and counsel victims of domestic violence and neglected or abused children. These patients are more likely to seek aid if their doctor recommends confidential and trusted counsel than if they have to seek help on their own. Working together, health care professionals, community groups, and legal advocates can help prevent these situations from escalating from an incident of abuse into a death or serious injury.

Potential solutions for domestic violence. Victims of domestic violence can request the following (for free)[42]:

- A restraining order to keep the offender away from their work, school, and home
- A move-out order for the offender and property control orders for cars, work tools, and other property necessary for self-support
- Child support and child custody orders
- The sheriff will serve the papers for free. Filing restraining order paperwork is free
- Payment for medical costs and property damages incurred because of the violence
- In some cases, asylum to ensure the patient cannot be sent back to the country where the violence occurred
- In some states, many of these protections apply to elders who are being abused by anyone (family member or nonfamily member)

Tips for domestic violence issues. Financial considerations are important and a lawyer can help the patient build a plan that addresses the complex needs of family violence victims. This means protecting the family home and property, addressing criminal law issues, and considering custody and support. These issues are complex, but are easier to deal with in a *civil proceeding* started by the parent than in a government proceeding started by the county's child protective services department.

Unmet Legal Need P: Planning for Advanced Care

Health-tie. The elderly, ill, and/or disabled are common victims of financial and physical abuse. Plans ensuring that an individual has someone they trust to care for them, watch over their assets, and keep an eye out for financial or physical abuse is a plan everyone needs, especially if they have limited assets and/or family.

Legal myth. "Estate planning is for rich people."

Potential legal solutions for advanced care planning:

- Advanced care planning can prevent evictions, protect family assets, and defend the patient from financial and physical abuse from non-relative caregivers.
- A *joint guardianship proceeding* allows a terminally ill, single parent to transfer custody of their children to another person before they die (ensuring they go to the right person).

- There are many probate proceedings that provide family protections for surviving spouses, dependent children, and disabled children that your patient may not know about. For example, a *petition for homestead*[43] enables a family to stay in a home until kids grow up, even if creditors or other heirs have a claim to it.
- If you are leaving assets to a disabled child, an attorney can set up a *special needs trust* to manage and protect his or her assets.[44]

Tips for advanced care planning issues. Families with limited assets and large debts may not think they can benefit from legal help. Spending a half-hour with an estate planning attorney may help them discover *survivors' benefits* and use *statutory protections* to keep limited assets safe from creditors.

HOW TO REFER PATIENTS TO LEGAL HELP

Helping a patient to understand the legal resources available to them can help them understand that the process may not be as difficult as it seems.

Referrals. For the purposes of this chapter, a referral to a legal consult means asking the patient to discuss his situation with a lawyer or social worker.

All patients may want to know the following:

- A legal consult is confidential
- Many lawyers will offer 30 minutes free and they may take the case on a contingency fee basis (they get paid from the litigation award rather than up front)

There are many sources to find an attorney:

- Lawhelp.org has contact information for state-approved legal referral services including the state and county bar associations. If the patient has a low income, Lawhelp.org has listings of free legal service in each state.
- Justhealth.info has legal information and resources for patients to educate themselves.
- Many areas have legal and social services information available by calling 211.

Table 6.2, organized under the IHELP categories, shows how to connect a patient to the best legal solution for their issue.

TABLE 6.2
Attorney Type Matching

Legal Need	Where to Start	When to Call a Lawyer	Type of Lawyer	Screening Questions
Income and Insurance				
Food	County welfare office	If an application for help is denied or benefits are suspended	Pro bono public benefits attorney (legal aid society)	Are there times during the month when you do not have enough food?
Utility protection or benefit programs	Contact utility company directly	If an application for help is denied or benefits are suspended	Pro bono public benefits attorney (legal aid society)	Have you applied for utility discounts based on your disability or family size?
Social security benefits Medicaid denial Medicare appeals	Local social security office	If an application for help is denied or benefits are suspended Questions if you qualify	Disability benefits attorney	Are there medical reasons why you are unable to work or go to school?
Medicaid planning	County welfare office	Call ASAP if planning to apply for Medicaid and have a spouse or kids	Elder law attorney, estate planning attorney	Are you concerned that the cost of your care may affect your ability to support your family?
Denied disability claims through private insurance company (employee benefit)	Human resources department	When you suspect your claim may be denied or has been denied	Disability lawyer	Have you missed treatments or appointments because of a denied insurance claim?

TABLE 6.2 (*Continued*)

Legal Need	Where to Start	When to Call a Lawyer	Type of Lawyer	Screening Questions
Housing				
Rental access	County welfare office	If an application for help is denied or benefits are suspended	Pro bono public benefits attorney (legal aid society)	Are you having any trouble finding or staying in adequate housing?
Eviction defense	Landlord	If a notice to quit has been served or there has been an eviction threat	Tenants' rights attorney; Landlord/tenant attorney	Are you having any trouble paying your rent or mortgage on time?
Habitability standards	Landlord, local housing authority	If landlord refused to remedy problem	Tenants' rights attorney; Landlord/tenant attorney	Do you notice any mold, mildew, or mice, or are there animals in the building?
Foreclosure defense	Mortgage company	If a notice to quit has been served or there has been an eviction threat	Real property lawyer	Did you know you may qualify for a mortgage reduction during a treatment plan?
Education				
Denied access for lack of documentation	School administration: principal and then school board	If enrollment is denied by the principal	Education attorney	Have you had any trouble enrolling your child in school?
Special needs— education plans and discipline issues	School administration: principal and then school board	If the school board refuses to test for special needs or sets a hearing for discipline	Education attorney	Is your child having trouble at school either academic or behavioral?

TABLE 6.2 (*Continued*)

Legal Need	Where to Start	When to Call a Lawyer	Type of Lawyer	Screening Questions
Employment				
Request changes to work environment	Employer	If the employer refuses to change the environment or the patient does not know what changes to request	Disability attorney Some employment attorneys	Are you having trouble with work because of a health condition, or are the responsibilities at work aggravating your health?
Unlawful discharge	Some state economic development agencies will hear complaints	If the employee suspects they might be fired or has been fired and wants damages for the lost wages and insurance	Employment attorney (plaintiff)	Do you have someone who is watching out for your employment rights and responsibilities?
Legal Status				
State policies on benefits	Anonymous call to county welfare office (they must provide interpreter, if present)	If benefits are denied, or the county welfare office response is not satisfactory	Immigration rights attorney Public benefits attorney	Free through local legal aid society, MLP, or immigrants rights organization
Personal and Family Security				
Domestic violence restraining order	Family law facilitator at local courthouse	If the case is complex or if the patient needs more help than the facilitator can provide	Domestic violence attorney Family law attorney	Are you afraid of any past and/or potential violence in your domestic life?
Child support	Department of child support service or family law facilitator	If the agency is not representing the patient's concerns	Family law attorney	Does the other parent of your child pay support and contribute to health care costs?

TABLE 6.2 (Continued)

Legal Need	Where to Start	When to Call a Lawyer	Type of Lawyer	Screening Questions
Spousal support	Family law facilitator	If the agency is not representing the patient's concerns	Family law attorney	Have you asked a court for spousal support?
Planning for Incapacity and Death/Probate				
Incapacity and death planning	State bar association may have sample forms	Most clients will use an attorney if they can afford one, and it is recommended if leaving assets outside of the family	Estate planning Attorney	Have you planned for the future? Who do I contact if you are too ill to speak for yourself?
Transferring guardianship of a minor	Local court may have packets of information or classes	Most clients will use an attorney if they can; court will have simplified forms for parents without attorneys	Probate attorney Guardianship attorney Family law attorney	Do you have a plan for your children?
Family protection from creditors	Local court may have packets of information or classes	Most clients will use representation if they can	Probate attorney if the person in debt is deceased Bankruptcy attorney if both spouses are still living	Are you concerned about losing your home or assets to creditors?

MEDICAL–LEGAL PARTNERSHIPS: A MODEL FOR SUCCESS

Even after receiving a referral for a legal consult, patients may be hesitant to find and speak with an attorney. MLP is a health care and legal services delivery model that aims to improve the health and well-being of vulnerable individuals, children, and families by integrating legal assistance into the medical setting. Forming an MLP is an effective method of increasing the number of patients who will ask for help because patients are more likely to speak with an attorney if the attorney is on-site and the doctor knows and recommends this service.

In 1993 Dr. Barry Zuckerman and one attorney, Joshua Greenberg, founded the MLPC to serve patient-families at Boston Medical Center. Over the course of the next 15 years, the program expanded into a national model for the delivery of health care. Lawyers—legal aid agencies, law schools, and *pro bono* attorneys—and front-line health care providers—doctors, nurses, and social workers—are now partnered at more than 225 hospitals and health centers nationwide, serving children, the elderly, patients with cancer, pregnant women, the formerly incarcerated, and other vulnerable populations.

The National Center for Medical–Legal Partnership supports the expansion, advancement, and integration of MLPs by providing technical assistance to partnership sites, facilitating the MLP Network, promoting leadership in law and medicine, and coordinating national research and policy activities related to preventive law, health disparities, and the social determinants of health.

MLP Outcomes

Cancer Patients Have Significant Nonmedical Needs

A recent study by LegalHealth, an MLP based in New York, found that the majority of cancer patients have unmet legal needs and legal intervention helped reduced their stress and worries. The study found that legal problems for patients with cancer are a *significant nonmedical need* that must be addressed to maintain quality of life during and after cancer treatment. Among the survey clients, 78% reported that having cancer created their legal difficulties. Legal interventions impact cancer survivors in the following ways:[45]

- 83% of the survey clients reported that legal services helped to reduce their worries and stress.
- 51% of the survey clients reported that legal services had a positive effect on their financial situation.
- 33% of the survey clients reported that legal services positively affected their family or loved ones.
- 22% of the survey clients reported that legal services helped them to keep medical appointments.
- 23% of the survey clients reported that legal services helped them to maintain their treatment regimens.

Legal Intervention Often Results in the Recovery of Funds for Both Patients and Clinical Facilities

Roswell Park Cancer Institute's partnership with Neighborhood Legal Services served 237 patients that were referred to the partnership in less than 3 years. The majority of cases involved permanency or custody planning and guardianships, advance care planning (health care proxies, powers of attorney, and wills), benefits advocacy (disability, insurance, or food stamps), estate planning, and housing. The attorneys also were able to obtain significant financial results[46]:

- Legal representation in 17 cases with complex insurance denials resulted in reimbursement to the hospital that totaled $923,188.
- In six cases, lawyers were able to win disability benefit insurance appeals. Some cases had significant retroactive benefits ($17,000, $11,000, and $4,000) and other cases resulted in award amounts of $600-$1,200 per month.

FROM PATIENTS TO POLICIES—ADVOCATING FOR SYSTEM CHANGES

The hands-on experience of health care providers is a very valuable social resource. What if the experience of your job or clinic (or that of another organization) shows that a change to its policies needs to be updated? Policy changes can help the enforcement of existing laws in a more equitable or effective manner. This is an important function of social development, both internally within your organization, and externally by working with other organizations and governmental agencies. As an example of a successful policy change, consider the story of Officer McGrath and Attorney Sprecher.[47]

In trying to protect victims of domestic violence, Officer McGrath routinely found that victims who were undocumented immigrants were hesitant to speak with police and testify against their abusers because they feared deportation. During the investigation of one of these cases, Office McGrath came into contact with a victim's immigration lawyer, Attorney Sprecher. Mr. Sprecher informed Officer McGrath that crime victims can apply for a special type of visa, called a U-VISA, if a police officer signs a certification stating the person was a victim and cooperated in the prosecution of the crime. Noting how this legal tool could inspire immigrants to testify, Officer McGrath issued a division-wide notice outlining the procedures for when the police personnel were authorized to sign the certifications. Since then, several crime victims received U-VISAs and the city council has adopted a resolution supporting the Police Department in using U-VISA certifications as a public safety tool.

In the midst of daily pressures, getting local law enforcement to change a procedure may sound like a colossal task. This example illustrates that when you come across an issue that matters, you can accomplish your objective by breaking down the process into manageable pieces:

1. *Identify the issue.* Start by giving credit to your frustration. The tip-off for the need for a policy change is a pattern of frustration. In the case above, the police officer notices a pattern of frustration about immigrant victims' refusals to testify.
2. *Identify the organization(s) that needs to change and who is in charge of the organization(s) (the boss).* One short-cut in finding the boss is asking the individual what his or her excuse is for not completing the requested action.
3. *Call the boss.* In the McGrath example, he was the boss and he still called his boss (City Council). More frequently than one might expect, a policy change only requires asking. For example, MLPs have had success in getting utilities companies to decrease the frequency with which they call and ask doctors to certify that their patients still have a disability.
4. *Give it another push.* If the answer from the first boss is no, then consider these four steps

    a. *Call the person (or their boss) three times.* Calling the person repeatedly, or sending letters, may get them to understand that this is a real issue that matters and needs to change.
    b. *Go up the chain of command.* If it is a local government agency that needs to change, calling your local city council member is a good way of inspiring change. For example, this author, Attorney Sarah Wessels, has personally had a government employee swear they could do nothing to accomplish the requested policy change and refused to discuss the subject. The requested change would allow a person with power of attorney to pick up birth certificates on behalf of an out-of-state resident who needed a copy immediately, usually for passport or visa issues. The Department of Health had a policy against allowing anyone other than the applicant to pick up the certificate. After a call to City Hall and a letter to the city attorney's office, the requested change happened in a week.
    c. *Complain to the media.* Many organizations have a sensitive public relations department, which means that even though they may not care about your issue, they may care about how the public perceives them not caring about your issue. Please see Chapter 5 on the best methods of contacting the media.
    d. *Punt the problem to another organization.* If you are not getting the results you want, you may consider building a team or handing the issue off to another person or organization. There are many

organizations that have full-time staff that are paid to spend their days making policy changes happen.

If you are not sure whom to contact about adopting your needed policy change, you may try the following:

1. Contact a health organization that works with the patient's health concern (such as the Autism Speaks organization for a patient with autism).
2. Contact a legal organization that works in the area of law (education rights or disability rights). Lawhelp.org has listings of nonprofit legal services organizations that you can search according to legal issue and geographic area.
3. Call an attorney who practices in a related area of law. Lawyers can be good teammates, not only because they study law but they may have financial or professional motivations to get involved, such as marketing publicity for their firm.

Nonprofit organizations can also be excellent teammates. Your clues that you will want to get an organization involved are as follows:

- You need a law or formal rule change
- You need money or funding (outside of your own funds)
- You need to file a lawsuit to get the change to happen

Getting an organization on board will be easier if you find one with a mission that is closely aligned with your cause. (See Chapter 9 for more on this topic.) For example, if you see a pattern of employee abuse (working unpaid extra hours, denied workers' compensation claims, etc.), look for an organization with a mission to protect employee's rights.

Handing the issue off to a legal organization is especially important if the problem requires some sort of *formal rule change*. Formal rules are developed by government agencies to clarify their policies to the public. These rules require a specific process that involves a "comment period" where members from the community can submit letters and a meeting where the agency will discuss the issues and make a decision. Legal organizations are set up to calendar when comment letters are due, who to send them to, and what legal language is required to get the committee, department, or organization to formally hear the complaint. The organization may ask that you submit a declaration in support. A declaration may sound complicated, but it is only a written statement of what has happened and why you think the policy change will be beneficial. If you care about the issue, submitting the declaration can be critical to accomplishing the change.

REFLECTION QUESTIONS

1. What legal myths or protections surprised you most?
2. What types of legal referral systems might be most helpful to patients seen in different types of health settings—community hospitals, urban private practice, and rural clinics?
3. Drawing on your personal experiences, what types of policy concerns have impacted your life or the life of a friend or family member? Identify possible solutions and who is in the chain of command.

PRACTICE MAKES PERFECT

1. What types of private information do you think you will be privy to in your practice? Consider the patients you have contact with. Which legal issues are mostly likely to be present?
2. How can you best become informed about community resources in your area? Is there a medical–legal partnership in your region? If so, find the closest one. If not, is there a social worker who is on staff to help with patient concerns? Identify this person and introduce yourself if you do not already know each other.
3. What types of policy concerns may complicate your practice? Identify whom you can reach out to for help.

NOTES

1. Federal Employers Liability Act 45 U.S.C. § 51 et seq. (1908).
2. 1956 amendments to Title II of the Social Security Act. 70 Stat. 815, 42 U. S. C. § 423 (1996).
3. Title XVI of the Social Security Act, as added, 86 Stat. 1465, and amended, 42 U. S. C. § 1381 *et seq.* (1982 ed. and Supp. V).
4. Social Security Act, 42 U. S. C. §§ 501–503 (1982).
5. Federal Government's Aid to Families With Dependent Children (AFDC) program established by the Social Security Act of 1935, 49 Stat. 620, as amended, 42 U. S. C. §§ 301–1394.
6. State programs are supported through Title IV—D of the Social Security Act, 42 U. S. C. §§ 651–669b (1994 ed. and Supp. II).
7. Federal Old-Age, Survivors, and Disability Insurance Benefits (OASDI) program, 42 U. S. C. §§ 401–431 (1970 ed. and Supp. V).
8. Retired Serviceman's Family Protection Plan (RSFPP), 10 U. S. C. §§ 1431–1446 (1976 ed. and Supp. IV).
9. General Assistance is provided by states under numerous public welfare codes, and example is Conn. Gen. Stat. Rev. § 17-2d (1965 Supp.).

10. Federal Food Stamp Act, 7 U.S.C. § 2019(d) (Supp.1976).
11. Low Income Home Energy Assistance Program, 42 U.S.C. § 8621–8630 (2008).
12. Sage, Adam. (2010). Patient-client stories. Retrieved from http://www.medical-legalpartnership.org/impact/patient-client-stories
13. Title XIX of the Social Security Act (SSA), as added, 79 Stat. 343, 42 U.S.C. § 1396 *et seq.* (2000 ed. and Supp. III).
14. Consolidated Omnibus Budget Reconciliation Act of 1985, 29 U.S.C. §§ 1161–1168.
15. Title XI of the Social Security Act (SSA) 42 U.S.C. 1315 *et seq.* (2010).
16. Medicaid Act 42 U.S.C. §1396(a)(10)(C)(i).
17. Medicaid Act 42 USC § 1396r-5; see also *Wisconsin Dept. of Health & Family Servs. v Blumer,* 534 US 473, 479 [2002].
18. Fair Housing Act, 42 U.S.C. § 3604(f)(3)(B) (2000). See also *Schuett Inv. Co. v. Anderson,* 386 N.W.2d 249 (Minn. Ct. App. 1986); *Whittier Terrace Assocs. v. Hampshire,* supra; *Majors v. Housing Auth. of DeKalb, Ga.,* 652 F.2d 454 (5th Cir. 1981); *Schuett Inv. Co. v. Anderson,* 386 N.W.2d 249 (Minn. Ct. App. 1986).
19. See *Pines v. Perssion* (1961) 14 Wis.2d 590 [111 N.W.2d 409]; *Lemle v. Breeden* (1969) 51 Hawaii 426 [462 P.2d 470, 40 A.L.R.3d 637]; *Javins v. First National Realty Corporation* (1970) 428 F.2d 1071 [138 App. D.C. 369], cert. den., 400 U.S. 925 [27 L.Ed.2d 185, 91 S. Ct. 186]; *Marini v. Ireland* (1970) 56 N.J. 130 [265 A.2d 526, 40 A.L.R.3d 1356]; *Kline v. Burns* (1971) 111 N.H. 87 [276 A.2d 248]; *Jack Spring, Inc. v. Little* (1972) 50 Ill.2d 351 [280 N.E.2d 208]; *Mease v. Fox* (Iowa 1972) 200 N.W.2d 791; *Boston Housing Authority v. Hemingway* (Mass. 1973) 293 N.E.2d 831.
20. Truth in Lending Act (TILA),15 USC §§1601–1667f (1994) enforced through Regulation Z (12 CFR pt 226); see also Home Ownership and Equity Protection Act of 1994 (HOEPA) (15 USC §§1647–1648; Pub L 103–325, 108 Stat 2160).
21. Tenant Based Assistance: Housing Choice Voucher Program, 42 USC § 1437f.
22. Truth in Lending Act (15 U.S.C. 1601 et seq.).
23. Discussed generally in *Pellandini v. Valadao,* 7 Cal. Rptr. 3d 413-Cal.: Court of Appeals, 3rd Appellate Dist. 2003.
24. Legal Aid of Nebraska (August 21, 2009), Medical–Legal Partnership benefits cancer patients, *Legal Aid of Nebraska Briefly.*
25. See generally *Hutchins v. Peabody,* 151 NH 82-NH: Supreme Court 2004.
26. Sage, Adam. (2010). Patient–client stories. Retrieved from www.medical-legalpartnership.org/impact/patient-client-stories
27. McKinney-Vento Homeless Assistance Act, 42 U.S.C. § 11381 *et seq.* and 24 C.F.R. § 583.100 *et seq.*
28. Individuals with Disabilities Education Act (IDEA or Act), 84 Stat. 175, as amended, 20 U.S.C. § 1400 *et seq.* (2000 ed. and Supp. V).
39. Americans with Disabilities Act, 42 U.S.C. § 12132.
30. Health hurdles: tackling legal barriers for kids (March 27, 2009), United Press International. Retrieved from www.upi.com/video/Features/2009/03/27/health_hurdles_tackling_legal_barriers_for_kids/UPI-12381694335209/.
31. Family and Medical Leave Act of 1993 (FMLA or Act), 107 Stat. 6, as amended, 29 U.S.C. § 2601 *et seq.* (1994 ed. and Supp. V).

32. Americans with Disabilities Act of 1990 (ADA or Act), 104 Stat. 328, 42 U.S.C. § 12101 *et seq.* (1994 ed. and Supp. V).
33. Americans with Disabilities Act of 1990 (ADA or Act), 104 Stat. 328, 42 U.S.C. § 12101 *et seq.* (1994 ed. and Supp. V).
34. Family and Medical Leave Act of 1993 (FMLA or Act), 107 Stat. 6, as amended, 29 U.S.C. § 2601 *et seq.*(1994 ed. and Supp. V).
35. Paid Family Leave Program of 2003, see generally Cal. Code Regs. tit. 22, §§ 3301(a)-1 to 3306(b)-1.
36. Esq. Cassie Springer-Sullivan (November 3, 2009), Adapted from training: insurance law, interacting with disabled clients, San Francisco: Springer-Sullivan & Roberts LLP.
37. Interim Guidance on Verification of Citizenship, Qualified Alien Status and Eligibility Under Title IV of the Personal Responsibility and Work Opportunity Reconciliation Act of 1996, 62 Fed. Reg. 61344 (November 17, 1997).
38. Personal Responsibility and Work Opportunity Reconciliation Act of 1996 (PRWORA) § 411.
39. Personal Responsibility and Work Opportunity Reconciliation Act of 1996 (PRWORA) § 110.
40. Immigration and Nationality Act ("INA"), 8 U.S.C. §§ 1158(a), 1253(h), and 1252(a) (1996).
41. 8 U.S.C. §§ 1228(b)(3) and 1252.
42. Violence Against Women Act of 1994, § 40302.
43. See generally *Casey v. Casey*, 109 P. 3d 345-Okla.: Supreme Court 2005.
44. Authorized by 42 U.S.C. § 1396p(d)(4)(A).
45. Randye Retkin, Julie Brandfield, & Cathy Bacich (January 2007), Impact of legal interventions on cancer survivors, *LegalHealth*.
46. Kerry J. Rodabaugh, Maureen Hammond, Dawn Myszka, & Megan Sandel (January 2010), A Medical-Legal Partnership as a component of a palliative care model, *Journal of Palliative Medicine, 13(1)*: 15–18.
47. Megan Sprecher & Michael McGrath (March 22, 2010), Op-ed: city of Cleveland takes an important step to ensure citizen safety," *Cleveland Plain Dealer*.

7

Class Action for Health Professionals

BRUCE L. SIMON AND THOMAS K. BOARDMAN

> *The class action was an invention of equity, mothered by the practical necessity of providing a procedural device so that mere numbers would not disable large groups of individuals, united in interest, from enforcing their equitable rights nor grant them immunity from their equitable wrongs.*
> —Montgomery Ward & Co. v. Langer, 1948

Imagine that a general practitioner in private practice discovers that one of the insurance companies she accepts has been routinely under-reimbursing her and delaying payments for services covered by her patients' health plans. Imagine that, upon further investigation, the general practitioner discovers that the reimbursements are only a few hundred dollars under the expected total. The general practitioner, like many, might feel she is now in a difficult position. On the one hand, she knows that she is being wronged by the insurance company. On the other, she worries that the costs of addressing her grievance might outweigh the possible return.

Imagine that a nurse employed by the a large private hospital group discovers upon closer inspection of her paystubs that her employer has been paying her overtime at a rate slightly less than one and a half times her hourly rate. Perhaps the employer's conduct, though systematic, has only resulted in the nurse's pay being docked a small fraction of her hourly wage. Similar to the general practitioner above, the nurse may believe that the effort and costs to bring a claim against the employer on her own may be too high.

These examples share a similar trait: a grievance that on an individual basis may be cost prohibitive to bring, but is emblematic of a common grievance, held by many. On this larger scale, the need to remedy the harm is more pronounced. For those who have not been a part of class action litigation before, the prospect of bringing a class action lawsuit may seem confusing and daunting. Hopefully, this chapter will dispel many of the concerns of those unfamiliar with the class action possess.

CLASS ACTION VERSUS INDIVIDUAL ACTION

> [A]ll persons materially interested, either as plaintiffs or defendants in the subject matter of the bill ought to be made parties to the suit, however numerous they may be. The reason is that the court may be enabled to make a complete decree between the parties, may prevent future litigation by taking away the necessity of a multiplicity of suits, and may make it perfectly certain, that no injustice shall be done, either to the parties before the court, or to others, who are interested by a decree, that may be grounded upon a partial view only of the real merits.—(West v. Randall, 1820)

History and Policies Behind Class Actions

In both of the examples in the introduction, the health professional that discovered the wrong might be hesitant to pursue litigation because she is concerned about the costs when weighed against the potential benefits. One of the elements of a class action that makes it unique is that typically the attorneys representing the plaintiffs do so purely on a contingency basis. In such an arrangement, class attorneys will front all of the costs associated with the litigation at no risk to the plaintiffs. Only if there is a verdict or settlement in favor of the class do the plaintiffs' attorneys get a fee. This allows individuals, like the hypothetical health care providers above, to take part in cases that can bring about systematic change regardless of whether their specific injuries amount to ten dollars or ten million. If an individual recognizes a wrong, large or small, that he or she shares with a larger group of people, the wrong is best corrected by a class action. The concept of a remedy for every wrong has been recognized by the Supreme Court and can be traced all the way back to Sir Edward Coke's scholarship on the Magna Carta (*Stoneridge Inv. Partners, LLC v. Scientific-Atlanta*, 2008).

Why a Class Action?

Claims brought as a class action differ from an individual action in how the complaint, the document filed with the appropriate court, is drafted. Unlike an individual action, where the plaintiff or plaintiffs bringing the claims represent only themselves, in a class action the plaintiffs named in the complaint ("named plaintiffs" or "class representatives") represent the interests of the entire class of people as defined in the complaint (the "putative class"). Put simply, in a class action a smaller group brings a claim to represent a larger group that shares similar traits. For centuries courts have allowed a few to bring claims on behalf of many in the name of justice and efficiency. In the name of justice even small harms deserve a remedy, and sometimes individuals must band together for the party at fault and public to take notice. Class actions are efficient for all parties involved because they prevent duplicative litigation. In the case of the general practitioner described in the first scenario, suppose the insurance company has tens of thousands of doctors under its plans and all of them were under-reimbursed. If class actions did not exist and all of the insured doctors each separately elected to pursue litigation, thousands of individual complaints would flood the defendant and the court with virtually the same factual and legal allegations.

HOW DOES A CLASS ACTION WORK, EXACTLY?

Class Certification

After a class action has been filed, the attorneys for the plaintiffs will file a motion to have the court approve the class as defined in the motion. This process is called "class certification." For a complaint to be maintained as a class action, the larger group that the smaller group seeks to represent must contain certain traits prescribed by the rules that govern civil lawsuits. Those rules are called the Federal Rules of Civil Procedure (Fed. R. Civ. P.) and the rule that primarily governs class actions is Rule 23. During class certification, the court applies the standards set out in Rule 23 to determine if the proposed definition is suitable for a class action and the named plaintiffs and their counsel are fit to represent that class.

Federal Rule of Civil Procedure 23
Numerosity. Under the Federal Rules, a putative class must be so numerous that it would be impractical for the court to join together all the separate cases in one large litigation. There is no minimum number of putative class members that will satisfy the numerosity analysis and several other factors such as geographic distribution, ability of each plaintiff to bring their own suit, and plaintiffs' financial resources influence whether the joining of individual cases would be feasible. However, numerosity is typically deemed met when there are at least 40 members of the putative class, but divisions have been certified for classes that contain less than 40 members and there is no magic number (*Consol. Rail Corp. v. Town*

of Hyde Park, 1995). Further, the numerosity analysis is context specific and courts must take into account the type of claims asserted, among other factors, as delineated in Fed. R. Civ. P. 23(a)(1) and *Gurmankin v. Costanzo* (1980).

If health professionals are experiencing an injury that they believe may be happening to others, they should contact a class action attorney with the basic information regarding their own experience and why they think the issue is pervasive. It is exceedingly rare for an attorney to charge any fee for an initial conversation or consultation. Further, any discussions with an attorney in anticipation of possible litigation are private and protected by attorney–client privilege. Similarly, with the advent of medical groups and the consolidation among such groups, a health professional could be a defendant in a class action lawsuit either by virtue of being part of a group that is sued or by being named individually. In that circumstance, it is advisable to contact an attorney well-versed in class actions, but typically the defense of such a case will only be done on an hourly basis. Those attorney fees should hopefully be covered by insurance, but not always.

Commonality. Next, a class petitioning to be certified must show that there are questions of law and fact common to all members of the putative class. Recently, the Supreme Court defined commonality as "requir[ing] the plaintiff to demonstrate that the class members have suffered the same injury. This does not mean merely that they have all suffered a violation of the same provision of law" (see Fed. R. Civ. P. 23(a)(2) and *Wal-Mart Stores, Inc. v. Dukes* [2011]). For a class to have sufficient common questions of law or fact, its claims "must depend upon a common contention—for example, the assertion of discriminatory bias on the part of the same supervisor. That common contention, moreover, must be of such a nature that it is capable of classwide resolution—which means that determination of its truth or falsity will resolve an issue that is central to the validity of each one of the claims in one stroke" (see Fed. R. Civ. P. 23(a)(2) and *Wal-Mart Stores, Inc. v. Dukes* [2011]). Thus, under this newly refined definition of commonality, the claims brought by the class must not only show that a common injury occurred to all (e.g., they were undercompensated by an insurance company), but that if the court ultimately finds in favor of the class, the remedy implemented to resolve that injury will have a common effect on the class (e.g., the court forces the insurance company to reimburse all undercompensated doctors).

Typicality. The typicality factor relates directly to the role of a class representative in a class action. The typicality prerequisite of the Federal Rules is fulfilled if the claims or defenses of the representative parties are typical of the claims or defenses of the class. Under the Rule's permissive standards, representative claims are "typical" if they are reasonably similar to those of absent class members; they need not be substantially identical (see Fed. R. Civ. P. 23(a)(3) and *Hanlon v. Chrysler Corp.* [1998]).

Adequate Protection and Representation. Federal Rule 23(a)(4) also requires that the class representatives must fairly and adequately protect the interests of the proposed class. Because all members of the putative class will be bound by the court's decision if the named plaintiffs prevail, the court must ensure that those not specifically named in the complaint are afforded adequate representation before the entry of a judgment that binds them (*Hansberry v. Lee*, 1940).

Typically, resolution of two questions determines legal adequacy: (a) Do the named plaintiffs and their counsel have any conflicts of interest with other class members, and (b) Will the named plaintiffs and their counsel prosecute the action vigorously on behalf of the class (*Hanlon v. Chrysler Corp.*, 1998)? In evaluating the first question, the court typically looks at whether the proposed class is divided into subclasses and, if so, whether those subclasses could have conflicting interests. For example, a case could have two subclasses, one that is only interested in prospective relief for the alleged wrong (e.g., an injunction prohibiting the injurious behavior), and one that asks for retrospective relief (e.g., monetary reimbursement). A situation could arise where the defendants wanted to settle the claim for retrospective relief, but the parties were still far apart on what the proper prospective relief is. In such a situation, if the same lawyers represented both subclasses then a conflict of interest may exist because the retrospective relief subclass wants to settle with defendants and secure the monetary relief, but the prospective relief subclass wants to fight on and get the best injunctive relief possible. If the court were to find that counsel representing both subclasses would have a conflict, the court has the power to assign different class counsel to each subclass.

Beyond the role of the attorneys and the potential for conflict of interest, the petition for class certification must show that the named plaintiffs are capable of fulfilling their duties as class representatives. The duties of a class representative are, among others, to:

- Hire competent counsel to pursue their claim.
- Review and approve the complaint as drafted by the attorneys before it is submitted to the court.
- Retain and search for documents that might be relevant to the case.
- Produce the documents when requested.
- Appear for a deposition if asked.
- Stay generally informed, through counsel and otherwise, of what is happening with the case.
- Appear at trial.

These requirements are in place to ensure the court that the class representatives, their counsel, and the relationship between the two are adequate to protect the interests of absent class members. Class representatives must satisfy the court that they, and not the counsel, are directing the litigation. To do this, class representatives must show themselves sufficiently informed about the litigation to manage the litigation effort (*Unger v. Amedisys Inc.*, 2005). However, the class representative is not a legal expert and is not required to have an encyclopedic knowledge of the case.

Predominance of Common Questions. Once a court finds that the proposed class action complaint, the class representatives, and their counsel all meet the four requirements of Federal Rule 23(a), the court must then turn to Federal Rule 23(b) to determine whether, given all the Federal Rule 23(a) factors, a class action and not individual lawsuits will be a superior method of adjudicating the claims. To make this decision, the court focuses on "the legal or factual questions that qualify each class member's case as a genuine controversy" (*Jackson v. Motel 6 Multipurpose, Inc.*, 1997).

Courts do not require that "[a]ll questions of law or fact...be common; but some questions must be common to the class and those questions must predominate over individual questions" (*Re HealthSouth Corporation Securities Litigation*, 2009). Even if shared experience and injury can meet the commonality requirement of Federal Rule 23(a), the standard for predominance of common questions of fact and law is more demanding (*Amchem Products, Inc. v. Windsor*, 1997). Predominance does not mean that all legal and factual issues are the same, but that most of them are. Slight differences in the legal claims among class members or a difference in the way their damages may be calculated will not usually preclude a class from being certified. Often, experts will be retained by class counsel to calculate damages, and one of the issues under the predominance standard is whether the methodology used by the experts to calculate damages is common to substantially cover all of the class members. Even courts and attorneys sometimes mix the commonality requirement with the predominance requirement. The simple way to look at this is that commonality requires that basically the same claims are being made for the whole class, and predominance is a more rigorous requirement that goes to the proof of the case by common evidence.

The reasoning of the predominance standard is similar to the above discussed requirements—to ensure that there are no conflicts of interest among putative class members and that the issues raised by the claims are not so disparate as to be more properly handled in separate trials.

Superiority of Case Management. To meet the predominance standard under Federal Rule 23(b)(3), the plaintiffs' counsel must demonstrate that a class action is the superior mechanism for the litigation. Factors relevant to this showing include: (a) the interest of the members of the class in individually controlling the prosecution or defense of separate actions, (b) the extent and nature of any litigation concerning the controversy already commenced by or against members of the class, (c) the desirability of concentrating the litigation of the claims in the particular court, and (d) the difficulties likely to be encountered in the management of a class action.

Appointment of Lead Counsel. Especially in large class actions, different groups of named plaintiffs may file class action claims in the same matter. Each different group of named plaintiffs will have its own attorneys. When the cases are filed, the court will appoint interim lead counsels to be the main contact point for the court and defendants. During the class certification processes, the court will appoint a firm, or group of firms, as lead (or co-lead) counsel for all of the named plaintiffs who filed claims, furthering the policy goal of efficiency because the court and defendants can direct their communications with plaintiffs through one source. Attorneys not selected as lead counsel will still be assigned to the case and able to advocate for their clients' needs, but they will do so under the direction of the lead counsel. Lead counsel are typically selected by the court based on the firm's prior experience in handling class action cases similar in substance and scale to the one the court is then certifying.

The Role of Class Counsel

> Beyond their ethical obligations to their clients, class attorneys, purporting to represent a class, also owe the entire class a fiduciary duty once the class complaint is filed.—(In re General Motors Corporation Pick-Up Truck Fuel Tank Products Liability Litigation, 1995)

Class representatives serve as the inspiration and driving force behind every class action. Without an individual's willingness to stand up and be involved to redress a harm, there would be nothing for the lawyers to do. Once the harm has been identified, hiring an attorney is one of the most important steps in the civil litigation process. Because of the unique characteristics of class actions, choosing the right attorneys to handle such complex litigation is of heightened significance.

The first act of any reputable class action attorney is to have a preliminary meeting with the prospective plaintiff to get the facts about the perceived injury. If the attorney believes the facts have merit, he will then conduct research about the laws that are meant to protect against the alleged injury and undertake a factual investigation. If both the factual and legal research show that there is a claim to be made against a defendant, the two parties will enter into a retainer agreement. The terms of the agreement will formalize the attorney–client relationship. As stated earlier in the chapter, all of the costs of litigation will typically be covered by the firm representing the named plaintiff. It should be noted that all attorney fees and costs awarded to the class action attorney must be approved by the court at the end of the case. This adds an extra layer of scrutiny to the fee agreement than would occur in a non-class case.

Once an agreement is in place, the law firm will draft a complaint. A complaint contains the facts and legal theories that the attorneys believe are best suited to redress the client's injury, based on their discussion with the client and their research. Assuming the client's injury was one believed to be experienced by many and thus proper for class action, the complaint will include provisions clearly stating that the plaintiff is bringing the complaint on behalf of all others similarly situated. It will also contain a preliminary definition of the class the named plaintiffs seek to represent. Before the complaint is filed with the court, the client must review the complaint to make sure he or she agrees with the facts and legal theories as stated by the attorneys.

The attorneys will then file the complaint with the proper court, usually the one closest to either the plaintiff or the defendant. The remaining procedural aspects unique to class actions are covered in the rest of this chapter.

Notice and Opting Out. In order for the class representatives to fairly and adequately represent the interests of absent class members, those class members not specifically named in the complaint must be able to object, opt out of the class, or otherwise ensure that their own rights and interests are protected (*Alberghetti v. Corbis Corp.*, 2010). Because any settlement or verdict that may occur later in a class action is binding on everyone covered by the certified class definition, once the court has certified the class the appointed counsel for the plaintiffs is required to inform the general public of the nature of the claims and the definition of the class through a published notice. Typically, notices are printed in widely read newspapers like the *Wall Street Journal* and trade periodicals specific to the industry subject to the litigation. Class counsel will also create a web page and advertise on the internet.

The notice must advise each putative class member that she/he has the right to exclude her-/himself from the action, become a class representative, or remain passive as an absent class member. The notice must also inform all putative class members that the judgment, whether favorable or not, will bind all class members who do not elect to opt out.

> To this end, the court is required to direct to class members the best notice practicable under the circumstances including individual notice to all members who can be identified through reasonable effort. We think the import of this language is unmistakable. Individual notice must be sent to all class members

whose names and addresses may be ascertained through reasonable effort.

(Eisen v. Carlisle & Jacquelin, 1974)

This notification is particularly important when the class action potentially involves the assessment of monetary damages. Imagine in the example regarding the hypothetical under-reimbursing insurance company that after the notice is posted, one of the largest private hospital companies in America (e.g., Hospital Corporation of America, HCA) that employed 50% of doctors covered by the insurance company elected to opt out of the class action. Assuming that under-reimbursement was roughly equal among all doctors, HCA opting out of the class would take approximately half of the monetary damages out of the class action case. If a party opts out of the class, it then has the option of bringing its own individual claim, negotiating with the defendants in private, or doing nothing at all.

There are certain types of cases, like employment cases, where class members have to opt in to participate in the class action. The notice procedures are essentially the same, but the class member has to affirmatively agree to be in the class, whereas in an opt-out class, if a class member just does nothing they remain in the class.

After the Class Is Certified. After the court certifies the class action, the case proceeds, for the most part, like a regular, individual lawsuit. Counsel for the class and for the defendants will file various motions and briefs in an effort to frame the case with the judge, and potentially the jury, in a manner that best fits their respective argument, but those motions will not differ significantly from the ones that would be filed in an individual case.

Of course, if facts and circumstances change, the parties defending the case may ask the court to redefine the class, narrow it, or decertify the class. Since the class action is a procedural device, it is deemed to be conditional and subject to modification even through the time of trial. If the class remains certified like most do, then any verdict and judgment in the case will bind the class members.

Resolution of the Case. Like most civil litigation, the vast majority of class actions do not go to trial. It is far more typical for both sides to agree on a settlement. Because class actions have the power to bind all members of the certified class that did not opt out, the courts must approve the terms of the settlement before it becomes official. Courts must approve any proposed class settlement to make sure that the terms are fair to all class members, even those who remained passive during the litigation and did not hire counsel. After the settlement is submitted to the court for approval, class counsel will send notice of the settlement and its terms in a manner similar to the one used to notice class certification. There will then be a time frame, similar to the opt-out period, when class members can file objections to the terms of the settlement with the court. The court will take any objections into account when making its final decision about whether to approve the settlement. Once the court approves the settlement, all remaining members of the class are bound by its terms. The same is true if a class action goes to trial and the jury returns a verdict in the plaintiffs' favor, as described above.

After final resolution of the case, either by settlement or verdict, the binding nature of class actions on all remaining class members means that no individual or entity that fits within the definition of the class as certified by the court can ever bring a claim against the defendants based on the same set of facts and legal theories. The fact that the settlement or judgment is binding in perpetuity to all parties is one of the foundational policy considerations of a class action. Instead of forcing plaintiffs and defendants alike to litigate countless repetitive claims, a single court can adjudicate all claims in a single case. Although the same primary elements of justice and efficiency run through all class actions, there are a wide variety of laws and statutes, referred to as "causes of action," that are appropriate vehicles for class actions.

Types of Class Actions

As important as understanding how class actions work is knowing under which cause or causes of action to bring a class action claim. Although the ultimate decision about which cause of action to bring a plaintiff's claims under is the attorney's, it is useful for the potential plaintiff to understand some of the legal protections he or she is afforded. Below is a simple, nonexhaustive list of statutes related to the health care profession that could be used as a vehicle for a class action. If these snapshots provoke further questions related to personal experience, please contact an attorney.

Examples of Causes of Action
Federal Statutes
Administrative Procedure Act: This Federal statute governs the ability of Federal administrative agencies to propose and establish regulations. The Act "permits suit to be brought by any person 'adversely affected or aggrieved by agency action'" based on a regulation or action of that agency (*Lujan v. Nat'l Wildlife Fed'n*, 1990).
American's With Disabilities Act (ADA): The ADA is essentially the Civil Rights Act applied to people with disabilities. It prohibits a wide range of discrimination based on a person's disability from employment discrimination to access to private and public buildings.

Electronic Communications Privacy Act: This act prohibits unauthorized government access to private electronic communications.

Federal Information Security Management Act of 2002 (FISMA): This act requires every Federal agency (e.g., Veteran's Affairs, Medicaid, Medicare, FDA) to have an agency-wide program for the security of information and information systems.

Genetic Information Nondiscrimination Act of 2008: This act prohibits discrimination based on genetic information in health insurance and employment. Under this act, insurers cannot deny coverage or raise premiums based on a genetic predisposition.

Health Insurance Portability and Accountability Act (HIPPA): This act was passed to allow greater access to health care by making employment-based health care more portable and easier to renew. It also attempts to curb insurance fraud and abuse creating broader protections for patients against insurers disclosing private health information.

Racketeer Influenced and Corrupt Organization (RICO): Although it is primarily thought of as a mafia-busting, criminal statute, RICO also provides private individuals harmed by a criminally corrupt organization the right to bring a civil suit for damages.

Statutes Related to Business (Such as Antitrust Statutes)

Sherman Act: The Sherman Act prohibits anticompetitive behavior in restraint of trade. This act was passed to break up monopolies around the turn of the 20th century. It prohibits such anticompetitive acts as price-fixing, monopolization, and attempted monopolization.

Clayton Act: The Clayton Act, similar to the Sherman Act, prohibits various anticompetitive behavior. It is primarily used to combat price discrimination by "curb[ing] the use by financially powerful corporations of localized price-cutting tactics which... gravely impair[] the competitive position of other sellers" (*F.T.C. v. Anheuser-Busch, Inc.*, 1960).

Note: Many states throughout America have their own versions of antitrust laws.

State Business and Consumer Protection Laws

California has arguably the most robust business and consumer protection laws in the country. These laws prohibit a broad range of conduct including, but not limited to, all unlawful, fraudulent, or unfair business practices, false/misleading advertising, contractual fraud, theft of trade secrets, interference with an economic relationship, and commercial defamation. Many other states have similar laws.

CASE STUDY: *KLAY V. HUMANA, INC.*, 382 F.3D 1241, 1274 (11TH CIR. 2004)

Plaintiffs: Physicians

Defendants: Aetna, CIGNA, Humana, Foundation Health, PacifiCare Health, Prudential, United, and Wellpoint

Allegations: Racketeering Influenced and Corrupt Organizations Act, Employee Retirement Income Security Act, and a California subclass for violations of California's Business and Professions Code § 17200 *et seq.*

A group of physicians brought a class action lawsuit against major health maintenance organizations. The named plaintiffs sought to represent a RICO and an (Employee Retirement Income Security Act) ERISA class. The RICO Class was defined as, "All persons in the United States (not including person insured by Medicare or Medicaid) who purchased or participated in health maintenance organizations, preferred provider organizations, and/or point of service plans, operated by [the respective insurance company] at any time during the period from October 4, 1995 through and the date hereof until [the company's] continuing illegal and wrongful conduct has ceased." The ERISA Class was defined as, "All persons in the United States who participated in ERISA-governed health maintenance organizations, preferred provider organizations, and/or point of service plans operated by [the respective insurance company] at any time during the period from October 4, 1993, through and after the date hereof until [the company's] continuing illegal and wrongful conduct has ceased."

The physician named plaintiffs sought to represent three classes. The Global Class was defined as, "All medical doctors who provided service to any person insured by any Defendants from August 4, 1990 to September 30, 2002." The National Subclass was defined as, "Medical doctors who provided services to any person insured by a Defendant, when the doctors has a claim against such Defendant and is not bound to arbitrate the claim." The California Subclass was defined as, "Medical doctors who provided services to any person insured in California by any Defendant when the doctor was not bound to arbitrate the claim being asserted."

The plaintiffs were physicians who were reimbursed by one or more of the defendant HMOs for treating patients covered by those HMOs. The plaintiffs alleged that the backbone of their relationship with the HMOs was that they would "be paid, in a timely manner, for the covered, medically necessary services they render." The physicians further claimed that the defendants systematically "deny, delay and diminish the payments due to [them]," and failed to disclose to the doctors that they were being underpaid. The complaint alleged that the HMOs' reimbursement systems were based on "covertly denying payments to physicians based on financially expedient cost and actuarial criteria rather than medical necessity, processing physicians' bills using automated programs which manipulate standard coding practices to artificially reduce the amount they are paid, and ... systematically delaying payments to gain increased use of the physicians' funds."

As articulated in the Second Amended Class Action Complaint, the plaintiffs alleged that the defendants' computer systems were programmed to systematically underpay the plaintiffs through a variety of methods:

- The systems were programmed to simply deny reimbursement for certain base codes that insurance companies felt were too expensive, notwithstanding their contractual obligations to both physicians and patients.
- When the systems read certain base codes on HCFA-1500 forms, they were programmed to interpret them as requesting reimbursement for less expensive procedures. This practice was referred to as "downcoding."
- The system was programmed to group certain base codes together, so that if the system reads certain combinations of codes on the forms, they will be interpreted as being only a single code, a.k.a., "grouping."
- The system was allegedly programmed to ignore certain modifiers that would drive up physicians' reimbursements.
- The system was designed to unnecessarily put their reimbursement claims in a "state of suspense before they are processed even though no additional information is needed or requested.... The end result is that average payment times exceed by multiples the time provided for by law in most states as well as the time set by contract and industry practice."
- The forms the HMOs send to physicians explaining the amounts of their reimbursements called "explanation of benefits" forms (EOBs) misrepresented or concealed the actual manner in which Plaintiffs' payment requests were processed so as to induce them to accept reduced payments.

The case originated when lawsuits were filed in four Federal judicial districts against Humana, Inc., for underpaying doctors in the manners described above. Later, a panel of judges decided to combine the suits against Humana with several other similar Federal suits from across the country filed against other major HMOs (*Re Humana Managed Care Litigation, 2000*).

According to the Opening Brief of Appellants Aetna et al. (p. 45), at the class certification stage the HMOs' primary defense was that "a single jury, in a single trial, should not decide the fate of the managed care industry." However, the Federal appellate court hearing the appeal from the lower Federal court's partial denial of class certification held that:

> We find such reasoning unpersuasive and contrary to the ends of justice. This trial is not about the managed care industry; it is about whether several large HMOs conspired to systematically underpay doctors. The issue is not whether managed care is wrong, but whether particular managed care companies failed to live up to their agreements. The plaintiffs are seeking nothing more than the compensatory damages to which they are contractually entitled, and the treble damages to which they are statutorily entitled.
>
> [I]f their fears are truly justified, the defendants can blame no one but themselves. It would be unjust to allow corporations to engage in rampant and systematic wrongdoing, and then allow them to avoid a class action because the consequences of being held accountable for their misdeeds would be financially ruinous. We are courts of justice, and can give the defendants only that which they deserve; if they wish special favors such as protection from high-though deserved-verdicts, they must turn to Congress.
>
> (*Klay v. Humana, Inc.*, 2004)

After the class certification was upheld by the appellate court, the case was sent back to the district court where it was again the subject of fierce litigation on both sides. By mid-2007, nearly all of the defendants had settled with the plaintiffs. The settlements; total value is well over a billion dollars and included sweeping changes to the HMOs' billing process. These mandated changes included:

- Implement a definition of medical necessity that ensures that patients are entitled to receive medically necessary care as determined by a physician exercising clinically prudent judgment in accordance with generally accepted standards of medical practice;
- Use clinical guidelines that are based on credible scientific evidence published in peer-reviewed medical literature (taking into account Physician Specialty Society recommendations, the views of physicians practicing in the relevant clinical areas, and other relevant factors) when making medical necessity determinations;

- Provide physicians with access to an independent medical necessity external review process;
- Establish an independent external review board for resolving disputes with physicians concerning many common billing disputes;
- Pay for the cost of recommended vaccines and injectibles and for the administration of such vaccines and injectibles;
- Not automatically reduce the intensity coding of evaluation and management codes billed for covered services;
- Ensure the payment of valid, clean claims within 15 days for electronically-submitted claims and 30 days for paper claims;
- Provide fee schedules to physicians;
- Establish a compliance dispute mechanism to address disputes regarding the Blues' compliance with the agreement; establish and/or maintain physician advisory committees; and
- Provide 90 days' notice of changes in practices and policies and annual changes to fee schedules.

(For more details, see www.hmosettlements.com/settlements/bluecross/BCBS-pressrelease.pdf.

CONCLUSION

Class actions have the potential to bring impactful changes to entire industries at little to no cost to the class representatives that bring them. They are a powerful and useful tool whereby a group of people with grievances that might seem individually insignificant can leverage their joint power as a class to achieve widespread remedies. Class actions also have a deterrent effect that may cause potential wrongdoers to think twice about their conduct because the stakes can be so high.

REFLECTION QUESTIONS

1. Aside from the above examples, what are some injustices that have occurred in the health profession that would be appropriate for a class action? Why?
2. What reservations might health professionals have about being a named plaintiff in a class action? What reservations are particular to the profession?
3. What characteristics of the above-discussed structure and procedure of class actions make them a good fit for health professionals? What features of the profession might make a class action less likely to be certified?

PRACTICE MAKES PERFECT

1. For a hypothetical class of patients or peers that has a harm in common related to your field of expertise, identify a class action attorney whom you could call.
2. Discuss the class action or individual litigation experience in general with a health professional who has been a plaintiff in a case.
3. Review privacy guidelines and laws before assessing if your patients might have a class action claim.

REFERENCES

Alberghetti v. Corbis Corp., 263 F.R.D. 571, 577 (C.D. Cal. 2010).
Amchem Products, Inc. v. Windsor, 521 U.S. 591, 623–624 (1997).
Consol. Rail Corp. v. Town of Hyde Park, 47 F.3d 473, 483 (2d Cir. 1995) (citing 1 Newberg on Class Actions 2d, (1985 Ed.) § 3.05).
Eisen v. Carlisle & Jacquelin, 417 U.S. 156, 173 (1974).
F.T.C. v. Anheuser-Busch, Inc., 363 U.S. 536, 543 (1960).
Gurmankin v. Costanzo, 626 F.2d 1132, 1135 (3d Cir. 1980).
Hanlon v. Chrysler Corp., 150 F.3d 1011, 1020 (9th Cir. 1998).
Hansberry v. Lee, 311 U.S. 32, 42–43 (1940).
Jackson v. Motel 6 Multipurpose, Inc., 130 F.3d 999, 1005 (11th Cir. 1997).
Klay v. Humana, Inc., 382 F.3d 1241, 1274 (11th Cir. 2004).
Lujan v. Nat'l Wildlife Fed'n, 497 U.S. 871, 913 (1990).
Montgomery Ward & Co. v. Langer, 168 F.2d 182, 187 (8th Cir. 1948).
Re Gen. Motors Corp. Pick-Up Truck Fuel Tank Products Liab. Litig., 55 F.3d 768, 801 (3d Cir. 1995).
Re HealthSouth Corp. Sec. Litig., 257 F.R.D. 260, 276 (N.D. Ala. 2009).
Re Humana Managed Care Litig., Nos. 1334, 1364, 1366 & 1367, 2000 WL 1925080, 2000 U.S. Dist. LEXIS 15927 (J.P.M.L. Oct. 23, 2000).
Stoneridge Inv. Partners, LLC v. Scientific-Atlanta, 552 U.S. 148, 180 (2008).
Unger v. Amedisys Inc., 401 F.3d 316, 321 (5th Cir. 2005) (citing *Stirman v. Exxon Corp.*, 280 F.3d 554, 562 (5th Cir. 2002); *Berger v. Compaq Computer Corp.*, 257 F.3d 475, 479 (5th Cir. 2001)).
Wal-Mart Stores, Inc. v. Dukes, 131 S. Ct. 2541, 2551 (2011).
West v. Randall, 29 F. Cas. 718, 721 (C.C.D.R.I. 1820).

8

Leveraging Research Findings: Learning the Practice of Advocacy

GERI L. DICKSON

If you do what you've always done, you'll be what you've always been.—Unknown

You, as a health professional, have the ability to change your practice and to advocate for change in providing health care for your patients/clients through the use of the research process. If you take the time to develop that inner "advocate" and begin the practice of advocacy, you will develop a different perspective on your profession. The practice of advocacy for change in professional practices begins by identifying a problem and then by answering the question: What if? To begin to answer that question and change policies by leveraging the data you collect, you will need to follow the traditional research process: identifying the problem, selecting the right research question(s), collecting data necessary to answer the question, analyzing the data, and presenting the research findings. The traditional method of disseminating findings is generally through publications in prestigious journals.

However, in the practice of advocacy, you must carry it one step further by disseminating the findings through invoking the political process with publications such as legislative testimony, editorials, OP-ED pieces and letters to the editor, press releases, and presentations at professional conferences, social networking, and any other possible means that can bring your research findings to light. It is also helpful in the design phase of the research, to ask those research questions whose answers will be most amenable to this type of publicity! Meanwhile, as a successful advocate for your patients, you must be prepared to safeguard patients' identity and autonomy, defend social justice, and inform as well as empower your patients to make healthier decisions.

Fulfilling the role of advocate by demonstrating what works better can serve as the basis for change in practice policies at the point of care, as well as standards of care at the level of professional organizations, or at the State or Federal levels, by changes in public policy. This chapter will provide guidelines and examples to enhance development of your inner advocate through an understanding of the research process, and the importance of research findings necessary to advocate for change at all levels of health policy development.

WHY DO RESEARCH?

Research might have sounded mind-numbing during your education, but answering questions that arise from your patient care and discovering answers that can be applied to enhance the quality of your health care practice can be exciting and bring about a new way of thinking and doing. Opportunities to evoke the practice of advocacy may abound in the newly reformed health care system (Affordable Care Act, ACA, 2010). Factors such as access to health care, as well as its cost and quality, will play major roles. As part of the reform, insurers will only pay for the outcomes of quality care, rather than for the numbers of procedures or visits by health care providers or even avoidable hospital readmissions. Moreover, there is a focus on patient-centered care where patients have access to their electronic medical records and are asked to participate in making major health care decisions. Online health care information and research findings are readily available, but it takes a certain amount of skill and means to access and evaluate such information. According to Johnson (2011), "the exponential progress made to date in the pursuit of electronic health platforms has the potential to further marginalize those populations who have traditionally been on the wrong side of health disparities" (p. e2). Research findings related to the key elements of the health care reformation can be leveraged to create change through the practice of advocacy at all levels.

This chapter provides the general guidelines to follow that will not only suggest how to think of advocacy through research, but also might make it more interesting for you. Leveraging research findings for advocacy may in the long run create policy changes that benefit your patients, save costs of care for the health care industry, and even improve the work environment for clinicians. Let us now explore the steps in the process of gaining the necessary evidence-based knowledge to leverage your research findings for policy change for the benefit of your patients.

IDENTIFYING THE RIGHT PROBLEM

Keeping people well or returning them to health, both mentally and physically, is the goal of all health practitioners. Evidence-based practices, based on research, are found in the literature of all health care disciplines and provide the basis for sound clinical decisions (Higa-McMillan et al., 2011; Hill, Alpi, & Auerbach, 2010; Mascia & Cicchetti, 2011; Swain, Whitley, McHugo, & Drake, 2010). Discussing "evidence" in a clinical context means optimizing your health care based on research or demonstrated best practices, rather than in a legal context in the sense of information that would tend to establish a "fact" (Nold & Bochmann, 2010).

Using data to leverage policies has a distinct advantage for your patients, but it also adds to your credibility among your peers and gains awareness of your work by health care stakeholders. Our patients need a great amount of help in order to change counterproductive health care policies; you can begin a research program that benefits a population of providers and receivers of health care alike. If you are in or are looking forward to an academic position, research may even be a mandate for you to maintain your faculty role.

It might take some searching to find the "right" problem that is likely to catch the eyes and ears of the news media, national professional organizations, health care providers, and/or consumers. Perhaps the idea is a different way of thinking about an old problem, something that would clearly demonstrate a new path forward. It also must be something that you are truly interested in and in which you are willing to invest time, thought, and energy in finding an answer to your question(s). At times, research questions can come from a problem that you or someone you know may have experienced; something of interest in which research findings could provide a new way of looking at a problem. Although clinical trials are considered a gold standard in research, the road there may start with a great thought about a possibility and begin with a much smaller study to get a handle on the problem.

Let us look at some examples of populations and problems that are ripe for advocacy. Elders are often not the most desired patients to care for, yet the life expectancy of our population is growing, particularly those over the age of 85. According to the 2010 census, 100-year-olds are no longer the novelty they once were. The elderly, by sheer dint of their political clout and staggering costs of caring for them, are a "problem" with immediate impact on policy makers. An advocate for this population could find many organizations with which to collaborate, but working with organizations is covered in greater detail in Chapter 9.

So, now that we have everyone's attention focused on the elderly, where could research be helpful? One area in which evidence-based practices have emerged is that of falls, particularly in our aged population

(Haines, Hill, & Hill, 2011). Patients may suffer immobility, fractured bones, decreased quality of life, and even death from severe falls. In this example, the problem is patient falls and the "what ifs" are the care practices for the prevention of patient falls. Data have shown that identifying the patients at risk for falls, assessing their potential for falls, and identifying practices more likely to prevent their falling can lead to fewer patient falls and the resultant problems. Patient falls, particularly among our elders, are a concern in all settings and researchers from many fields have developed practices that demonstrate how to decrease the number and severity of falls (Haines, Hill, & Hill, 2011; Nod & Bochmann, 2010). Our growing cohort of elders is a segment of our population for which advocates are sorely needed to enable elders to live out their lives with the highest degree of dignity and quality possible.

Following the money in health care, significant resources are devoted to the care of hospitalized or long-term care patients. An area ripe for the practice of advocacy is safety of patients, particularly in regard to costly and harmful medication errors. This problem area has also been studied by many disciplines (Flitcroft, Gillespie, Salkeld, Carater, & Trevena, 2011; Gimenez, Zoni, & Rodriques, 2011; Schnipper, 2011; Weetman, Coombers, & Bionardi, 2010). The interdisciplinary medication processes involve physicians, pharmacists, and nurses; knowledge of the patient is as important as knowledge of the drug. Inpatients, as well as today's outpatients who could wind up as tomorrow's inpatients, need to be taking the correct medications. In these days of poly-pharmacy and the not infrequent use of prescribed medications as recreational drugs, surveillance of patients taking prescribed medication would seem to be more necessary than ever before.

But can surveillance actually help? If an outpatient is not adhering to the routine for a particular drug or drugs, it takes some investigating to determine the reason or reasons, and here is where research may come to the aid of advocacy efforts. Specifically, research could explore the best practices for monitoring of patients to help them adhere to a drug regimen.

On the inpatient side of the equation, nurses are the key personnel in the administration of medication and are the best source for knowledge about the patient and the drug. Nurses prevent twice as many medication errors from reaching the patient as do physicians and prevent three times as many errors than pharmacists (Rothchild et al., 2005). A stressful environment and many patients to care for sometimes interfere with best practices for successful drug administration. Interruptions and distractions in hospitals during nurses' medication administration have been identified as a major problem. Interdisciplinary teams of physicians, pharmacists, and nurses are working together to find out what and how to reduce medication errors (Propp et al., 2010). Lawsuits alleging wrongful death due to medication errors can be costly, so you can be sure that advocacy efforts backed by careful research in this area will attract attention.

As you have gathered from these examples, what works or not in practice is the genesis of a research problem to collect data to discover evidence-based solutions to common problems, which, in turn, can be addressed by using your practice of advocacy at the point of care. Problems and issues can arise from any source and at any time around certain agendas and with a different population of people, particularly in marginalized population groups. Your task is to find the right problem for you and your peers. Together you can address specific viewpoints related to a problem with an interdisciplinary care team, plus specific members' input. Remember, keep the focus on the practice of advocacy for change in health policies at all levels by leveraging research findings.

WHAT IS GOING TO BE BIG NEWS?

Most research requires funding; even small studies may have a cost with time involved to seek IRB approval, collect data, analyze data, and disseminate results. Therefore, keep in mind that the issues that are important today in the health care system are the ones that most likely will engage key stakeholders and legislators in supporting your findings. One way to identify current health care issues or problems is to look into what proposals are being called for by the National Institutes of Health (NIH). You can find current NIH calls for proposals, as well as older ones and funded research, on the net (http://grants.nih.gov/grants/guide/search_results.htm?year=active&scope=not). For a foundation that supports health care research, look up the Robert Wood Johnson Foundation website (www.RWJF.org). Spending some time on these websites may inspire, as well as give you a heads-up as to what research is important today.

One issue ripe for research and advocacy is the implementation of health care reform. For example, providers are scrambling to establish Accountable Care Organizations, hospitals are looking to hire physicians, and providers are searching for ways to provide quality of care and means by which to convert to electronic records. All of these are big news items, and are stressed in the proposed reforming of our health care system (ACA, 2010). Another strong issue, associated with the above, is ways to care for marginalized populations in providing quality care at a reasonable cost. There is some evidence to support employing advanced practice nurses, especially those with a Doctor of Nursing Practice (DNP), to provide quality primary care to patients (Eapen, Reed, & Curtis, 2011).

Dr. Jeff Brenner, a New Jersey physician, has documented his leadership in developing interdisciplinary community teams to increase care and reduce costs in the poorest areas in Camden, New Jersey. With the use of interdisciplinary teams led by Advanced Practice Nurses and community workers, they fill human needs and provide primary care (Gawande, 2011). Dr. Brenner has developed the Camden Coalition, without a physical clinic, which depends totally on street corner and home visits. Importantly, as only one outstanding outcome, the Camden Coalition has been able to save the city $3.5 million by improving the health and reducing the emergency room and hospital visits of just one patient (Gawande, 2011). Brenner's success is data based, beginning with New Jersey data from the Dartmouth Atlas that led to the expanded database he has introduced that allows Camden, New Jersey, physicians to view laboratory results, radiology reports, emergency-room visits, and discharge summaries for their patients from all the hospitals in Camden. These data not only demonstrate cost patterns but also doctor visits and hospital admissions—an idea whose time has come. Just imagine the potential cost savings and increased quality of patient care (Gawande, 2011).

In a similar vein, the prevention of hospital readmissions of heart failure patients is a good example of developing ways to save financially, as well as to increase the quality of care. Some hospitals have implemented transition programs in which advanced practice nurses remain in close contact with patients via phone, in person, or in telehealth visits to ensure that their medications are taken as prescribed and that the patient's weight is stabilized, both important in managing congestive heart failure.

Manning (2011) presents a model of transitional care that suggests nurses, with advanced education, could help improve the self-management of patients with congestive heart failure, which in turn reduces hospital readmissions. Stauffer et al. (2011), in a randomized controlled trial of congestive heart failure patients, reported a 48% reduction in 30-day hospital readmissions rate in the treatment group, who received transitional care with advanced practice nurse led teams. Naylor, Aiken, Kurtzman, Olds, and Hirschman (2011) reported in their review of the literature only nine studies that reported positive data regarding the readmission of the heart failure patient. These studies were difficult to compare because of varying degrees of methods and rigor, and some were focused mostly on economic savings (Naylor et al., 2011). However, Stauffer et al., in a recently published study, reports a higher rate of reduction in 30-day re-hospitalization than do some of the earlier studies (Coleman, Parry, Chambers, & Min, 2006; Naylor et al., 1999; Peikes et al., 2009). Although all of these treatment plans were nurse led, the management plans varied as did the readmission rates. However, they all reported reductions in readmissions at 30 days, which then continued to decline at 60 days and 90 days after hospitalizations.

Although this is an important area, the researchers would need to follow a similar research design for hospitalization rates to be compared. The management model proposed by Manning (2011) might be a beginning, but the selection of participants along with the size of the sample and the data collected (patients vs. records) must be the same for comparison's sake.

These are some areas that are garnering major attention. However, what area of health care really excites you? Women's care; disparities in health care; care of our elders, immigrants, children; genetic issues; hospital readmissions; end-of-life care; and so on? You can choose, but be sure to gather the facts so you can use your research findings to leverage that cause, and transform health and health care for your patients.

ASKING THE RIGHT QUESTION(S)

After identifying a newsworthy problem, the next step in the research process is developing a research question(s) in an area in which you are interested. Questions that can be answered by a yes or no are not useful research questions. Research questions must lead to evidence that determines data-based answers rather than a yes or a no. For example, a research question might be developed that says "Does monitoring reduce patient recidivism?" which leads to a yes or no answer. However, this is not a research question that would provide useful research findings or that would tell you what is important in monitoring patients in order to prevent relapse in their disease or health status. Instead a research question such as "What has an impact on preventing patient recidivism?" would provide some substantive data to address how and what kind of monitoring would prevent disease relapse in patients or increase activities that might jeopardize their health.

You also want to keep in mind that you are not soliciting opinions, so "should" or "could" are not appropriate words to begin a research question. Another idea to think through when designing a research question is to start with a question that is neither too broad nor too narrow. Evaluating the previous research on your topic can help to firm up a research question, or perhaps you can think in terms of small research steps to get the answer to a broader question.

In continuing with the concept of evidence-based practice, Mascia and Cicchetti (2011) conducted a study exploring "the extent to which social relationships can affect physician's attitudes toward evidence-based" (p. 798). As little is known about this topic, a goal, instead of a research question, of the study was identified as "To what extent are physician characteristics and inter-physician professional relationships associated with their attitudes and evidence-medicine implementation?" (p. 799). This beginning has the ability to become known by professional organizations, which in turn could change medical care at the point of care.

In a study in the field of education, a discipline where more work has been done regarding teaching methods, the following research questions were developed: (a) Do experienced elementary teachers in 1967, 1987, and 2007 have different purposes for asking students questions? and (b) Are there differences among today's experienced and inexperienced elementary and secondary teachers regarding what they think are the most important purposes for asking students questions? (Wallace & Hurst, 2009, p. 3). Presenting the findings from such a question in a manner that lay people can understand might be interesting to the press or legislators with today's emphasis on teaching methods and teachers' competencies.

But before actually finalizing a question or purpose of a study, a literature review is in order. A medical library or the website for PubMed (www.ncbi.nlm.nih.gov/pubmed) will give you access to a diverse array of journals; you will need to set up filters to relate to your specific problem. In doing the literature search, you may also find that someone else has solved the problem, but the findings have not yet become common knowledge. You may still want to use that research question to see if your results are comparable to the literature, keeping in mind that one study does not set the standards; many studies are needed to develop strong evidence for best practices. If you know you are planning to advocate for this issue, then the research serves as a point of discussion or debate to begin the practice of advocacy.

Other considerations include checking to see if the scope of information necessary to do this research is available to you. You will need to identify the participants in your study who will answer your research questions. Are they available to you? Do you have access to the type of data that you need to answer your research question? Do you have the necessary time to address adequately this question? After you have designed your study, you will need to seek approval from the Institutional Research Board (IRB) of the agency where you propose to do the study or the agency that is supporting you. Bear in mind that several categories of potential research participants need special approval, such as children or adults who are not able to make their own decisions about voluntarily taking part in this research. Most importantly, exchanging ideas with your colleagues and refining your research questions are useful in this iterative process.

Additionally, often you may begin to collaborate with other stakeholder organizations to include a secondary analysis of the data they might already have collected. For example, in developing a demand forecasting model for nurses in New Jersey, we were able to use data collected by the American Hospital Association. They had already collected national data annually of the numbers of nurses per patient day in hospitals, which we could use to forecast the future demand for the nurse workforce in New Jersey. Oftentimes some organizations may have a wealth of data, but not the time or the expertise to analyze it. For example, Lustig, Kureshi, Delucchi, Iacopino, and Morse (2008) used data that Physicians for Human Rights had on hand to make the point that medical evaluations of asylum seekers were helpful in court. Alternatively, these organizations may be helpful in collecting data that the rest of us would have a hard time accessing. For example, in a different study, Lustig partnered with the National Association of Immigration Judges (NAIJ), which was instrumental in corralling their membership to participate in a survey in judicial burnout. Without NAIJ's help, the study would have been far less successful (Lustig, Delucchi, Tennakoon, et al., 2008; Lustig et al., 2009). Giving thought to the means to collect data that will lead to findings of great interest to the public media may often lead to building relationships with formal organizations.

SELECTING THE RIGHT ANALYTIC METHOD

Your knowledge of research methods, or your availability to work with more advanced research partners, is also a consideration in finalizing the research question. For example, are you prepared to survey participants by developing an adequate instrument that will provide the data you need to seek advocacy for your participants? Or are there instruments already developed and available (some at a cost) that you can use to answer your research question? Are these instruments in a language and writing style that your participants will understand to answer appropriately? Or would a method that allows you to interview and record patients' responses for later analysis be a better choice for this research? Qualitative methods, which use words as data, are effective when little is known about the topic from participants' perspectives.

Once you have your research question(s) clarified and have identified the sample of the population you will be studying, the next step is deciding on a research method that is congruent with your research question. For example, a "what" research question may frequently be addressed by qualitative methods. Qualitative methods use words, instead of numbers, as their data. The particular types of methods for qualitative research include, but are not limited to, narrative analysis, case studies, grounded theory, phenomenology, hermeneutics, and some forms of content analysis. Specific journals, for example, *Qualitative Health Research,* only publish qualitative research. Research books also are available; some may focus on your particular discipline, but a good starting point is *The Qualitative Researcher's Companion* (Huberman & Miles, 2002).

Scale item surveys and secondary data analyses use quantitative methods that require statistics to answer the research question(s). These research questions generally begin with "why" or "how," rather than with the "what" of qualitative research questions, although sometimes "what" questions are also appropriate for descriptive quantitative measures. Statistical analysis is based on the concepts of probability and central tendencies (mean, median, and mode). Some questions can be addressed by using descriptive statistics to analyze and present the research data from "what," "how," or sometimes "why" questions. Data from more complex questions and large sample sizes may require sophisticated statistics designed for large studies to identify causal relationships or predictive factors of "why" things are happening. For a refresher on basic probability and statistics you can consult a free online text book that reviews these concepts (www.statsoft.com/textbook/elementary-concepts-in-statistics/?button=1). Many other statistics textbooks are also available with advanced methods.

For more sophisticated statistics, you will most likely need a biostatistician as a partner. Medical schools and universities generally have statistics departments and you may be able to find a mentor/collaborator within those settings. For relatively simple questions involving modest amounts of time, academically based statisticians will often help on condition of inclusion as authors on published results in peer-reviewed journals. Checking academic journals for articles in your focus area is another way you might find a mentor for more complicated studies.

SUMMARIZING FINDINGS

When all is said and done, you will need to present your findings in relation to your research question(s) in a logical, reasonable way for your readers to understand what you found. The findings should be straightforward and clearly demonstrate what you found and any surprises you might have encountered. The findings, for example, may be presented in the form of a story or a table of findings in qualitative research, while in quantitative findings a table (see Table 8.1), or a bar graph (see Figure 8.1), or a pie chart (see Figure 8.2) is most compelling. Both qualitative and quantitative research findings may be depicted with a schematic, as shown in Figure 8.3.

Which of these graphical depictions would you use to make the point that seven times as many cases occur among 55-year-olds

TABLE 8.1
Tabular Presentation of Incidence of Disease X by Age

Age	Incidence/100,000	Total Cases (%)
25	113	4
35	247	8.8
45	683	24.3
55	792	28.2
65	591	21.1
75	381	13.6
All	2,807	100

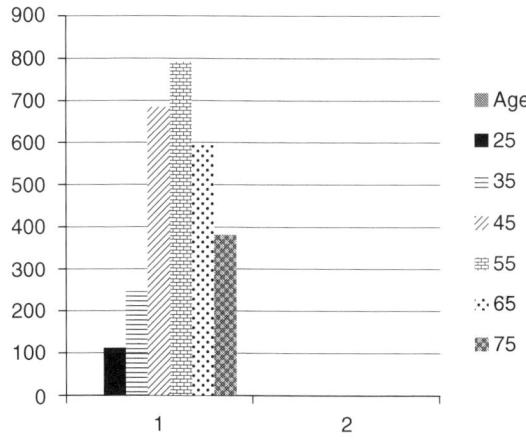

FIGURE 8.1
Bar Graph Showing Incidence of Disease X by Age

compared to 25-year-olds? What if you wanted to show that more than half of all the cases occurred among people aged 45 and 55? Or if you wanted to show the total disease burden (number of cases) across all ages?

In addition, in your written presentation, you will discuss the findings one by one, clearly, in the text. You will also include any limitations to your study, as well as where you are going from here (e.g., identify the next research step or the partners you will need to advocate for your population). Most importantly, as an advocate, you will present your findings in the best manner to help persuade others of a necessary change for health policy at the point of care, the professional organizational level, or in the public policy level.

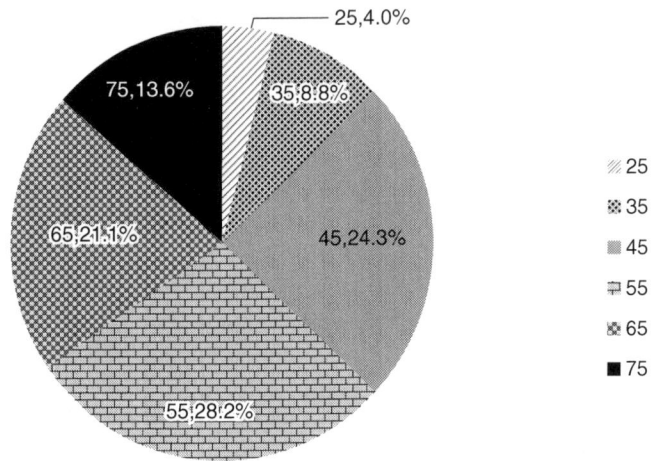

FIGURE 8.2
Pie Chart Showing Percent Distribution of Disease X by Age

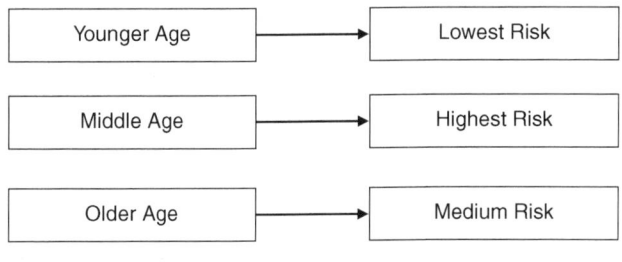

FIGURE 8.3
Risk of Disease X as a Function of Age

CASE STUDY: A QUALITATIVE METHOD STUDY OF SCHOOL COUNSELORS

In this study by Singh, Urbano, Haston, and McMahon (2010), the *problem* identified was that many school counselors did not practice advocacy at all levels in their school systems. Their *research question* was: "What advocacy strategies do school counselors who self-identify as social justice advocates use to enact change within their school communities?" (Singh et al., p. 16). Thus, these researchers developed a *grounded theory* study to examine this question. Following the grounded theory methodology of Corbin and Strauss (2008), they developed interview questions for self-identified counselors who practiced system-wide advocacy. Recursivity was built into each stage of the research and data from the interviews were analyzed as each interview was conducted; some were face-to-face and others were by phone. Consistent with grounded theory, data saturation was reached (i.e., no new data were forthcoming) with the fourteenth interview and two more were then conducted for a total of 16 interviewees. The codes and results were shared with all the researchers and agreement for validity of the findings was reached by member-checking, which is sharing the findings with some of the participants to check if they agreed with the initial findings.

The *findings* consisted of seven overarching themes: "(a) using political savvy to navigate power structures; (b) consciousness raising; (c) initiating difficult dialogues; (d) building intentional relationships; (e) teaching students self-advocacy skills; (f) using data for marketing; and (g) educating others about the school counselor role as advocate." The findings were used "to support the further integration of advocacy competence in school counselor training, practice, and scholarship" (Singh et al., 2010, p. 144). They then explained each theme in depth and prepared an emerging model of social justice strategies that school counselor advocates used in making system changes (p. 138).

This qualitative research clearly identifies the basics in the practice of advocacy and resulted in changes in university programs for school counselors to include advocacy and justice in their curricula. The findings were publicized through the journal article and meetings of counselors. The participants in this study were identified as experienced advocates for social justice, so they already had made changes in their school systems. As one participant said, "I think that first you advocate, and then if you have time you do the other things. But whether it's on a small scale, or whether it's with a specific student, or with a particular population within the county, that's our number-one role" (Singh et al., 2010, p. 141). Typical of grounded theory study, quotations of the participants and how they implemented social justice in their school systems were published to bring to life the overarching eight themes. Thus, these themes were shared with other counselors, and mentoring was provided to assist new graduate counselors in becoming advocates for their students and to provide social justice within the school system. Last, but certainly not least, a course was developed in the school counseling program that emphasized and shared how experienced advocates had implemented the practice of advocacy.

CASE STUDY: RESEARCH FINDINGS USED TO ADVOCATE FOR EXPANDING THE NURSING WORKFORCE

Part 1–Setting the Stage

Nursing workforce shortages have plagued nursing since it became a profession that required certification through licensure in the first decade of the 20th century. However, the most recent shortage, beginning in the late 1990s to early 2000s, has lasted longer and was more intense than earlier shortages. In 1995, the Robert Wood Johnson Foundation (RWJF) put out a national call for states to gather data for the demand and supply of the nurse workforce in their states in order to develop strategies to educate an adequate supply of Registered Nurses (RNs) that meet the needs of patients. New Jersey was one of the 20 states awarded a 3-year so-called "Colleagues in Caring (CIC)" grant and then a 3-year renewal grant (1996–2002). Each state had a lead agency and in New Jersey it was the College of Nursing in Rutgers, the State University of New Jersey. Substantial collaboration was built among diverse groups of nurse educators, administrators, and healthcare stakeholders. A nurse demand forecasting model and method for collecting supply data were developed during the project and laid the foundation for further research regarding the New Jersey nurse workforce.

In order to continue our work, building on the attributes decided by the collaborative started during the CIC project, we decided to follow the direction of the "grandmother" of all nurse workforce centers, the North Carolina Center for Nursing, funded by a line item in the University of North Carolina budget since 1991. Although New Jersey legislation established the New Jersey Collaborating Center for Nursing on December 12, 2002, no financial appropriation was tied to the legislation (N.J., P.L., c116). Research findings in hand regarding the future supply and demand for nurses, we began to establish collegial relationships with stakeholder organizations with active legislative lobbyists, such as the New Jersey State Nurses Association, the Health Professional and Allied Employee (AFL-CIO) union, and the New Jersey Hospital Association. Next, we met in small groups with individual legislators, such as the chairs of the Assembly and Senate Health Committees, the Chairs of the Education Committees in both houses, the Chair of the Ways and Means Committee, and our individual legislative representatives. Eventually, we garnered the support of some legislators in both the State Senate and the Assembly to advocate for funding to maintain the Center. We tried to leverage our research findings regarding the predictive nurse demand model for nurses in New Jersey: Our forecasts indicated a double digit shortfall in 2006 (which did ultimately occur). Unfortunately, although a bill was introduced to create a line item in the Rutgers, the State University of New Jersey, budget, the bill died in committee. However, with these collaborations built and consistent research findings, we, in New Jersey, laid out a strategic funding plan that would provide basic operating costs for a New Jersey Center for Nursing and moved ahead with our strong collaborative partners and evidence-based studies.

Part 2–Descriptive, Quantitative Findings and an Executive Summary

Easily understandable numerical data, along with poignant narrative data, can be particularly evocative. Policy makers love personal stories, and the composite of the descriptive data were chosen to elicit the kind of answers that lend themselves well to advocacy. The executive narrative summary, developed from the descriptive findings, made a compelling case for how the safety and quality of New Jersey health care was in jeopardy. In 2005, the New Jersey Center for Nursing established a partnership with the Center for Health Outcomes and Research Center at the School of Nursing, University of Pennsylvania, to participate in a multiple-state survey of RNs in New Jersey, Pennsylvania, Florida, and California regarding the staffing and workload of patients as correlated with patient outcomes. The carefully designed survey was fielded along with a letter on the Board of Nursing stationery and signed by the presidents of the Board and the Center. In New Jersey, we received data from 24,206 RNs from a random sample of 50% of all actively licensed RNs in New Jersey. Our 50.5% response rate might sound low to a peer-reviewed journal, but we were able to point out in our advocacy efforts that participants comprised about 25% of the actively licensed New Jersey RNs workforce! The sample provided a wealth of descriptive data of the composition of the New Jersey RN workforce, as well as contributed to the collaborative larger study (Aiken et al., 2010).

    A comprehensive report, *The State of the New Jersey Nursing Workforce in New Jersey: Findings from a Statewide Survey of Registered Nurses*, addressed the following: "What are the characteristics of the typical New Jersey nurse? What are the challenges that New Jersey nurses face during their work day?"

(Flynn, 2007, p. 6). The report was released initially at an educational conference of the Center, funded by a grant from the New Jersey Health Initiatives of the RWJF. The report was then distributed widely among legislators and health care stakeholders. These descriptive data from the study, such as the number of nurses present in the current workforce and the number that are expected to leave over the next two decades because of retirement, were then used by the Center staff to demonstrate what the future would hold for the health care system in New Jersey, without an adequate professional nurse workforce. Now take a look at the "Executive Summary" which compellingly and succinctly embodies the findings as the work life of an average New Jersey nurse. Supported by the statistics, this story drives the point home by being an emotionally gripping, important contribution for the practice of advocacy. The entire report is housed on the New Jersey Center's website (www.njccn.org/pdf/Flynn_Survey_Report.pdf).

The "average" RN licensed in New Jersey is a 50-year-old woman who works more than 10 hours a day. But many, if not most, days she feels that her patient workload prevents her from taking even a 30 minute meal break.

She has more than 24 years of nursing experience and considers herself a proficient to expert nurse. Yet she has concerns that her patient workload is sometimes so high that it will cause her to miss an important change in a patient's condition. Sadly, she is also concerned about the nursing care that her patients needed during her workday but that she was unable to provide due to time constraints and not enough staff. She is frequently exposed to patient complaints and verbal abuse. She feels little support from her manager and despite her experience and skills she rarely receives recognition when she does a good job. She is teetering on the brink of emotional exhaustion.

Yet, despite these obstacles she maintains a sense of personal accomplishment. She knows that she makes a difference in her patients' lives.

Her challenge is to keep her patients safe and her mental health intact during the long and difficult workdays.

Our challenge is to create systems, processes, and environments that support her in her important work (Flynn, 2007, p. 5).

Part 3–Leveraging These Research Findings in the Practice of Advocacy for Patient Care

Now, how did we leverage these findings and the educational capacity data the Center has collected annually since 2003 to advocate for operating funds to sustain the Center and its important work? We started our action plan in April 2007 by scheduling a Policy Forum in the State House in Trenton. At the Forum, we presented data on both the nursing workforce and on the educational capacity of New Jersey nursing schools—the supply pipeline. A panel of nursing leaders from practice and education, as well as a representative from the Department of Labor, responded with their reactions. An active discussion followed the presentation and the panel responded to a magnificent State House room packed with three legislators, many legislative aides, nurse leaders, and other health care stakeholders.

Immediately after the Forum, we met with the Senate Health Committee Aides and representatives of the New Jersey State Nurses' Association, the major nursing lobbying organization in New Jersey. As public employees, we can educate about an issue or problem, but not lobby. This was the beginning of a process that resulted in a law being passed requiring that 5% of all New Jersey initial and renewal RN and LPN licensing fees were allotted to the Center each year (N.J., P.L., 2009, c47). Depending on the number of licensees, the funding may vary slightly from year to year, but amounts to about $400,000 per fiscal year. This law also placed the Center within the College of Nursing, Rutgers.

To recap, the work of the CIC program laid the initial research ground work and support for the legislation. Then, the professional publication of a report of the research findings, the State House Forum, the widespread distribution of the report, the personal contact with legislators and other stakeholders, the presentation of the findings at nursing meetings, the support of the major nursing organizations and nurses were all ways of leveraging the research findings to implement and support legislation that would allot funds for the Center. A front-page article in a statewide paper featuring the findings of the report also helped to provided leverage. The Center's purpose, from the legislation, is to "function as a future-oriented research and development organization that will develop and disseminate objective information and provide an ongoing strategy for the allocation of State resources directed toward the nursing workforce, which will assure the best possible nursing care for the residents of the State" (N.J., P.L., 2002, c116, p. 1).

Baby boomers have turned 65 in 2011, with an estimated 7,000 becoming eligible for retirement every day. The huge numbers of retiring nurses, coupled with the aging of the general population, produces a "perfect storm" for a nurse shortage. So, we continue to focus on the nurse workforce and related research. A survey is being fielded now on a sample of New Jersey RNs between the ages of 50 and 70 to investigate what factors influence nurses to retire, as well as what incentives employers might implement to encourage experienced nurses to stay. These data will be useful to employers to develop a phased retirement plan for each institution, along with incentives and new roles for the older, experienced nurses to contribute their practice wisdom.

LESSONS LEARNED FROM USING RESEARCH FINDINGS IN HEALTH CARE ADVOCACY

From working with the State legislators and occasionally with our representatives at the national level, we would like to share some valuable lessons we learned about leveraging our research findings to advocate for policy change.

- **Speak and write in bullet points**. Legislators, especially at the State level, may have other jobs and all are very busy learning about all the many professions, diseases, environmental toxins, and so on that need to be addressed by turning issues into laws. When issues come up they need to have information on the details to understand the problems and to decide how to vote. In our experience, most of the legislators or aides like to listen to facts that are clearly outlined from an expert perspective, which beats reading tomes of research-based literature. It is your job as an advocate to make your points clear with examples and a summary handout made up of bullet points of facts leading to conclusions.
- **Get to know the legislative aides**. As described in Chapter 4, they have direct access to the legislators and will gather information, impressions, and perspectives on a particular issue. They are usually young, bright, and very influential in getting their legislators to make decisions.
- **Put politics aside**. Regardless of your political persuasion, when approaching a legislator or aide, put partisan politics aside and present your research findings in a way that persuades the legislators to agree with your points to benefit his/her constituents.
- **Educate with "just the facts."** Most likely if you are a State employee or are the benefactor of foundation funding, you will not be able to lobby. Therefore, you role is to educate the legislative decision makers. *Never* say "vote for legislation S123." A fine line distinguishes lobbying from educating a legislator about your research findings.
- **Respond to all requests to testify on your particular issues**. No matter how busy or how tired you might be, do your best to respond to all requests to speak about your issue. If you are absolutely unavailable,

then send a representative in your place or send written testimony, which will be distributed.
- **Be prepared**. Do your homework so you can answer any questions that may come up. If you do not know the answer, do not fudge, but say something to the effect of "I will get more information and get back to you."
- **Listen carefully**. Do not take center stage, but, rather, listen carefully and take your clues from the people to whom you are listening. This is a great way to gather new ideas and put forth "words of wisdom."

These are some useful specifics we found helpful in developing our inner advocates. You may be able to add more to the list.

CONCLUSION

With the new knowledge gleaned from this chapter, hopefully you will be able to awaken your inner advocate and begin to have an impact on health policy at the point of care, at the professional organizational level, or at the public health care policy level. Evidence-based practice and policy development are no longer the purview of medicine alone. Many other professionals, such as nutritionists, nurses, physical therapists, health educators, mental health practitioners, and many others, are now involved in advocating for health policy change, and it is work that strengthens all of us. Harking back to the quotation at the beginning of this chapter, if you have been able to learn how to do things differently, you will move beyond what you've always been.

REFLECTION QUESTIONS

1. As a health professional, what credentials and experience would be helpful to mention to others as you use research findings (either your own or those of others) to advocate?
2. How can you best present complex research findings in ways that are understandable to legislators who do not have training in healthcare?
3. What are the general requirements of a research proposal for the Institutional Review Board (IRB) in your institution?

PRACTICE MAKES PERFECT

1. Imagine the research findings you would like to have in hand to advocate for a cause of interest to you. What study would be ideal to conduct in order to reach that conclusion?

2. Choose a healthcare issue that really resonates with you and develop a "fact sheet," using research evidence to support your position. (As you prepare to keep an appointment with a legislator, you must know who they are, what committees they are on, what their positions are on your issue, and how you can touch their inner advocate.) Now, write a follow-up letter with that advocacy issue and identify the next steps.
3. Choose a research article, either a qualitative or quantitative study, and write a "story" using the findings of the study. Discuss with your peers whether or not the story was helpful in understanding the findings.

REFERENCES

Aiken, L., Sloane, D., Cimiotti, J., Clarke, S., Flynn, L., Spetz, J., Seago, J., & Smith, H. (2010). Implications of California nurse staffing mandate for other states. *Health Services Research, 45,* 904–921.

Coleman, E. A., Parry, C., Chalmers, S., & Min, S. J. (2006). The care transitions. *Archives of Internal Medicine, 166*(17), 1822–1828.

Corbin, J., & Strauss, A. (2008). *Basics of qualitative research* (3rd ed.). Los Angeles, CA: Sage.

Eapen, Z., Reed, S. D., & Curtis, L. H. (2011). Do heart failure disease management programs make financial sense under a bundled payment system? *American Heart Journal, 161*(5), 916–922.

Flitcroft, K., Gillespie, J., Salkeld, G., Carater, S., & Trevena, L. (2011). Getting evidence into policy: The need for deliberative strategies? *Social Science & Medicine, 72*(7), 1030–1046.

Flynn, L. (2007). *The state of the nursing workforce in New Jersey: Findings from a statewide survey of Registered Nurses.* Newark, NJ: New Jersey Collaborating Center for Nursing.

Gawande, A. (2011). Medical Report: The hot spotters: A solution for health care's costliest cases. *The New Yorker, January 26,* 40–52.

Haines, T. P, Hill, A., & Hill, K. D. (2011). Patient education to prevent falls among older hospital inpatients: A randomized controlled trial. *Archives of Internal Medicine, 171,* 516–521.

Higa-McMillan, C. K., Powell, C., Ki'l, K., Daleldeń, E. L., & Mueller, C. W. (2011). Pursuing an evidence-based culture through contextualized feedback: Aligning youth outcomes and practices. *Professional Psychology, Research and Practice, 42*(2), 137–144.

Hill, E. K., Alpi, K. M., & Auerbach, M. (2010). Evidence-based practice in health education and promotion: A review and introduction to resources. *Health Promotion Practice, 11*(3), 358–366.

Huberman A. M., & Miles, M. B. (2002). *The qualitative researcher's companion.* Thousand Oaks, CA: Sage Publications.

Gimenez, M. A., Zoni, A. C., & Rodriques, R. C. (2011). Developing a programme for medication reconciliation at the time of admission into hospital. *International Journal of Clinical Pharmacy, 33*(4), 603–609.

Johnson, M. O. (2011). The shifting landscape of health care: Toward a model of health care empowerment. *American Journal of Public Health, 101*(2), 265–270. doi/10.2105/AJPH.2009.1898

Lustig, S. L., Delucchi, K., Tennakoon, L., Kaul, B., Marks, D. L., & Slavin, D. (2008). Stress and burnout among United States immigration judges. *Bender's Immigration Bulletin, 13,* 22–30, 43–47.

Lustig, S. L., Karnik, N., Delucchi, K., Tennakoon, L., Kaul, B., Marks, D. L., & Slavin, D. (2009). Inside the judges' chambers: Narrative responses from the National Association of Immigration Judges Stress and Burnout Survey. *Georgetown Immigration Law Journal, 23,* 57–82. Retrieved from https://articleworks.cadmus.com/geolaw/zs900109.html

Lustig, S. L., Kureshi, S., Delucchi, K., Iacopino, V., & Morse, S. (2008). Asylum grant rates following medical evaluations of maltreatment among political asylum applicants in the United States. *Journal of Immigrant and Minority Health, 10*(1), 7–15.

Manning, S. (2011). Bridging the gap between hospital and home: A new model of care for reducing readmission rates in chronic heart failures. *Journal of Cardiovascular Nursing, 26*(5), 368–376, 379.

Mascia, D., & Cicchetti, A. (2011). Physician social capital and the reported adoption of evidenced-based medicine: Exploring the role of structural holes. *Social Science & Medicine, 72,* 798–805.

Naylor, M. D., Aiken, L. H., Kurtzman, E. T., Olds, D. M., & Hirschman, K. B. (2011). The importance of transitional care in achieving health reform. *Health Affairs, 30*(4), 746–754.

Naylor, M. D., Brooten, D., Campbell, R., Jacobsen, B. S., Mezey, M. D., & Paul, M. V. (1999). Comprehensive discharge planning and home follow-up of hospitalized elders: A randomized clinical trial. *JAMA, 28*(7), 613–620.

Nold, A., & Bochmann, F. (2010). Examples of evidenced-based approaches in accident prevention. *Safety Science, 48,* 1044–1049.

Peikes, D., Chen, A., Schore, J., & Brown, R. (2009). Effects of care coordination on hospitalization, quality of care, and the health care expenditure among Medicare beneficiaries. *JAMA, 301*(6), 603–618.

Propp, K. M., Apker, L., Zabava Ford, K. W. F., Walllace, N., Serbenski, M., & Hofmeister, N. (2010). Meeting the complex needs of the healthcare team: Identification of nurse-team communication practices perceived to enhance patient outcomes. *Qualitative Health Research, 20,* 14–28.

Rothchild, J. M., Landrigan, C. P., Cronin, J. W., Kaushal, R., Lockley, S. W., Burdick, E., & Bates, D. W. (2005). The critical care safety study: The incidence and nature of adverse events and serious medical errors in intensive care. *Critical Care Medicine, 33,* 1694–1700.

Schnipper, J. L. (2011). Medication safety: Are we there yet? *Archives of Internal Medication 171*(11m), 1019–1020.

Singh, A. A., Urbano, A., Haston, M., & McMahon, F. (2010). School counselors' strategies for social justice change. A grounded theory of what works in the real world. *Professional School Counseling, 13*(5), 135–145.

Stauffer, B. D., Fullterton, C., Fleming, N., Ogola, G., Herrin, J., Stafford, P. M., & Ballard, D. J. (2011). Effectiveness and cost of a transitional care program for heart failure: A prospective study with concurrent controls. *Archives of Internal Medicine, 171*(14), 1238–1243.

Swain, K., Whitley, R., McHugo, G. J., & Drake, R. E. (2010). The sustainability of evidence-based practices in routine mental health agencies. *Journal of Community Mental Health* (46), 119–129.

Wallace, R., & Hurst, B. (2009). Why do teachers ask question? Analyzing response from 1967, 1987, and 2007. *Journal of Reading Education, 35*(1), 39–46.

Weetman, T., Coombes, I., & Bionardi, G. E. (2010). Reducing medication errors. *Lancet, 375,* 461–462.

9
Working With Families and Community Organizations

ROBERT HENDREN AND LEE GROSSMAN

*The community stagnates without the impulse of the individual.
The impulse dies away without the sympathy of the community.—*
William James (1842–1910)

One of the most important and essential components of effective advocacy is forming successful coalitions. Multiple, diverse voices speaking a similar message is louder and more compelling than a single voice from one constituency. The combination of family and community groups with health care professionals is becoming a powerful and effective force for improving health facilities, creating relevant programs, and being awarded funding from legislatures, government agencies, private foundations, private and public insurance companies, and philanthropists.

In this chapter, we describe why families and communities form organizations and why you, as a health professional, should collaborate with them. We describe the challenges inherent in these collaborations and develop an approach for health professionals to seek out and cultivate mutually beneficial partnerships that advance a common cause. Throughout the chapter, we will illustrate our points with case studies that showcase successful collaborations.

PARENT/FAMILY ORGANIZATIONS AS PARTNERS—WHY DO THEY FORM?

Welcome to the culture of parent/family organizations! Health professionals first need to understand why organizations comprised of families and other community members form in the first place. Reasons include:

- Desire to have a support network
- Raise awareness for a particular cause
- Support and develop a particular service or intervention
- Fund programs
- Drive advocacy efforts
- Move research forward

By forming an organization, family members and other interested community members can capitalize on the advantages of involving as many like-minded individuals as possible while providing a structure to make the group sustainable and productive (Hoagwood et al., 2010).

Parents and family members are primarily motivated to start and maintain these organizations by their deep dedication to those loved ones with a significant health issue and their passion for helping them and others affected by the same condition. Many of these parents also believe, and in most cases justifiably so, that the communities that they reside in are lacking in the appropriate services and supports for their families. As a result, they will start an organization to deliver such services or fill a void that is not available in their communities.

What Are the Benefits of Collaborating With Family and Community Organizations?

Clear benefits from collaborating with family/parent groups may not be obvious prior to a successful collaborative experience, and health care professionals may feel ambivalent about entering into a partnership. While some professionals may believe that their concern is justified by the potential compromise of the office-based relationship between the professional and the patient and his or her family, many professionals who have had the experience of this broader collaboration are appreciative of the fact that the context of the family is vitally important and involvement of the entire community surrounding the family often leads to the best outcomes. Professional partnerships with family organizations leads to deeper appreciation of the importance of caregiver stress, the presence of health care disparities, and issues of access to services that affect health outcomes (Ochoa & Nash, 2009).

Enhanced persuasiveness is another reason that the experienced health care advocate will be motivated to collaborate with family organizations. Going alone as a professional to visit a legislative aide or to address the legislature or a potential funder can give the appearance that the concern is really a "guild" issue and the professional or professional organization is motivated by self-gain. Going as part of a collaboration between mental health providers and families brings the strength of both perspectives: that of the family's very personal experience with an illness, and that of the professional and/or the professional organization about what is clinically necessary.

Successful collaborations can bring great success and pleasure. We recall many occasions where a group cheer and group hug followed the passage of an important piece of legislation or the end of an obstructive or discriminatory rule or regulation. However, there are many challenges. Sometimes the family members may believe that professionals do not have the time to listen to their stories or concerns. Sometimes the professional may feel they have to listen to long-winded, individual "war stories" from a family member when they already know the issue. Sometimes perspectives about what is really important may be quite different.

CASE STUDY: FORMATION OF THE AUTISM SOCIETY OF AMERICA

In 1964, Dr. Bernard Rimland published *Infantile Autism: The Syndrome and Its Implication for a Neural Theory of Behavior,* which presented a biological and neurological basis to autism and was a contradiction to the prevailing theory on autism at that time: that it was caused by a psychological detachment between the child and the mother. As Dr. Rimland's book became popular, he was inundated by letters from families around the world that agreed with his theories. Again and again, families expressed a sense of disconnect from the service community, lamented the lack of support, and highlighted their solitary struggles to help their children cope with autism.

As a result of these letters, in 1965 Dr. Rimland invited his correspondents to attend an organizational meeting at which the Autism Society of America was founded to lend support to families and individuals with autism, advocate for lifespan services, and raise awareness.

The collaboration among families and a health professional in this case study is similar to others you will hear about from many other family advocates. For many illnesses and disabilities, families have felt compelled to organize their own nonprofit associations to obtain the assistance that they feel is lacking. We are aware of numerous stories and reports detailing the financial and emotional problems and the self-sacrifice that family members endure to create and maintain their organizations. In spite of these hardships, most of the advocates believe that their cause and work is too important to give up, and they have few or no regrets for their collective efforts and the energies exerted. The commitment they have to the cause and their affected family member makes them among the greatest advocates for the condition they represent.

It is important to understand that the parent/family organizations and their advocates bring with them a sense of urgency to their cause as they believe that every day without adequate or appropriate services is another day that makes the life of their loved one more difficult. The families typically experience a great deal of stress through their constant dealings with the condition or disease. Most of the parent/family organizations see the value in collaborating with other organizations, government entities, professionals, and the community as a whole. The cause they represent is generally much larger than what they can serve and involves the engagement of multiple associations. These collaborative efforts include fundraising, awareness, providing or receiving services, educating the public and/or professionals, seeking media attention, advocacy, supporting elected officials and agencies, working with foundations, engaging the government at all levels, and supporting or advocating against various legislation.

HOW DOES THE HEALTH PROFESSIONAL FIT IN?

Community organizations recognize the added benefits that are associated with a close working relationship with the professional community. In general, health professionals bring the credibility of medical science to an organization and its cause. Health professionals have a strong interest in the issues represented by the organization, perhaps because of their specific research expertise or perhaps because they themselves may have family members with the illness or disability. Whether health professionals participate as other members do or serve in an advisory role, their sharing of cutting-edge information is highly valued by the group. Additionally, the group derives a psychological benefit from the presence of a health professional; he or she can help group members feel validated, understood, and cared about by at least one member of the health care community.

That said, health professionals looking to connect with a community organization should keep in mind potential causes of a group's hesitation to collaborate. Many of these parent/family organizations were started as a result of members' perceptions about a lack of appropriate services and supports available to their individual family member or cause. Some of the family advocates may believe that government agencies and/or health professionals are not interested or have other motives for not providing the services to their family member. This suspicion can result in skepticism about what a health professional would add to the group. For example, families may worry that the professional will continue an office demeanor of being the authority whose professional opinion is always correct and thus not fully appreciate the broader family and community perspective.

Health professionals seeking to start or connect with a community organization should understand that many of the advocates become "experts" in the condition they represent. Through their own exposure of caring for a person with a disease or disability, spending countless hours researching the latest news reports, and networking with others to share timely and relevant information, family members' knowledge of the condition becomes not only invaluable for their loved ones' well-being, they become authoritative on the subject of the condition as well. The success of the relationship between an advocate and a professional and/or government agency is often dependent upon mutual respect. Additionally, the recognition of success of the service provided to the individual with the condition is often directly related to the perceived collaborative effort that exists between the advocate and the servicing agent. The strength of these collaborations with medical professionals can positively affect how family members perceive services their loved ones receive.

HOW TO IDENTIFY AND APPROACH A COMMUNITY ORGANIZATION

If, as a professional, you want to become involved with a family or community organization, you will generally find a receptive audience. Associations usually want to engage with the professional community and welcome their involvement. As a professional, be sure that the group aligns with your values and philosophy in treatment and services so as to find an appropriate fit. This perspective often can be learned by speaking with the association's leadership, attending and observing at the support or membership meetings, and reading their materials. There are several ways to enter the organization but it is usually beneficial to know someone in the organization who can provide an introduction. This can be a family member that you treat or have treated, another professional who works with the organization, or a representative that you meet at a community event. They have an opportunity to get to know your style and endorse it and you have someone to provide you with some insights to the structure and the membership of the organization. You might attend a meeting before offering to become more involved or your contact may invite you to speak or meet with the leadership. It is usually desirable to enter the meeting with the participants feeling that you have an appreciation of the organization. If you are entering the organization as a professional it is fine to identify yourself as such but you may also say something personal such as "I have a deep appreciation of the importance of the good work your organization is doing." If you also have a family member who has a condition that has increased your appreciation of the organizations work you should mention this when you feel comfortable, as it often helps break down assumptions. Once a fit is determined, becoming involved can occur through volunteering, being a part of their professional advisors, or offering to be present at meetings. This interaction can be very rewarding to the professionals and the volunteers, and both can gain positively from the collaboration.

> **CASE STUDY: BILL OF RIGHTS FOR CHILDREN WITH MENTAL HEALTH DISORDERS AND THEIR FAMILIES**
>
> We were both part of the children's mental health coalition that ultimately created a "Bill of Rights for Children with Mental Health Disorders and Their Families," despite initial controversy over a key word (www.aacap.org/cs/root/resources_for_families/patient_bill_of_rights). The ongoing coalition consisted of the American Academy of Child and Adolescent Psychiatry (AACAP), the Autism Society of America (ASA), the Child and Adolescent Bipolar Foundation (CABF), Children and Adults with Attention-Deficit Hyperactivity Disorder (CHADD), the Federation of Families for Children's Mental Health (FFCMH), Mental Health America (MHA), and the National Alliance on Mental Illness (NAMI). The Bill of Rights represents the standard of what families living with mental illnesses should expect from treatment. The Bill of Rights was created because of the inconsistency of accessible mental health care services throughout the country.
>
> A major impediment to reaching an agreement between the professional and the family organizations was this sentence: "Treatment must be family-driven and child-focused. Families and youth, (when appropriate), must have *a* primary decision-making role in their treatment." Historically, both professionals and families have wanted to have *the* primary decision-making role. Families felt that this point was essential to receiving treatment tailored to their family and their child. Professionals worried that relinquishing this role might compromise the quality of treatment in which they would want to participate. The debate was resolved by the highlighted

"a" in the statement. This phrase says that the family will have a primary decision-making role but it implies that others such as the provider will have a shared decision-making role as well. This compromise satisfied both groups and supported the collaborative role increasingly recognized as essential to effective, quality health care.

Now That They Want You, How Do You Collaborate With Community Organizations?

Too often professional organizations and family/parent organizations do their work in isolation from each other. Sending information from one organization to the other may be a first step. Professionals can share health information with community organizations either individually or in tandem with their own organizations. This might include "Fact Sheets" from related professional organizations, interesting professional publications, and research studies. If the studies are complicated, a brief discussion of the scientific issues can help the findings be accessible and useful to the family organizations.

A next step can be to develop educational programs and materials together. Just as professional conferences can benefit from a parent on a conference planning committee, professional presenters at family conferences can discuss such topics as parenting tips or an educational review of therapies or disorder-specific presentations. A health professional can help draw a broader audience. Presentations by one group to the other benefit from having planning meetings in advance to tailor the presentation to the audience. The creation of educational materials also benefits from the combined perspective.

As the collaboration develops, fundraising for common goals are often more effective when professionals and family members prepare a strategy and do the "asks" together, as described in Chapter 10. Writing grants to regional and national foundations should have the perspective of the consumer and the provider. Presentations to prospective philanthropists are more compelling when planned and executed together.

Identifying potential legislation that professionals and family members mutually support or oppose can lead to an effective strategy for collaboration. For example, the AACAP has an annual advocacy day for children's mental health. Families from around the nation come to Washington, DC, during a national meeting of child and adolescent psychiatrists. The AACAP office of government affairs arranges visits to key legislative aides for family–professional teams. "Advocacy Day" begins with a briefing of the important issues and key talking points about why the legislative office should support or not support the bill are presented verbally and in a short fact sheet. A similar approach has been taken effectively at several State legislatures. Both partners report great satisfaction and a number of important bills have been successfully supported or blocked.

Developing new programs when a need is identified is yet another way that families and professionals can successfully collaborate. Insurance reform, respite care, special school programs, resource centers, new facilities in needed locations, integrated treatment facilities at schools, primary care offices, and community-based organizations are examples of programs amenable to successful collaborations focused on their development.

Avoiding Problems in Collaborations

Collaborations and coalitions generally fail because the expectations of all parties are not articulated, the effort and reward of the parties can appear to be disproportional and the time frame for success is not defined. As described in Chapter 3, the most auspicious of collaborations are those formed by various parties who come together for a unique and limited purpose benefitting all collaborators who are willing to forego individual gain. If all are willing to proceed under these terms and with clear expectations of the responsibilities involved, then a collaboration has a greater chance of succeeding.

It is important for all parties to draw up an agreement about who will do what, according to what specific timeline, and by which steps to accomplish the task. Equal attention must be given to who will serve in various leadership capacities. Regardless of the outcome, all should anticipate sharing equally in the results. Mutual respect and trust among all the parties is paramount; the success of these efforts is dependent on an unwavering level of cooperation and diligence. On the contrary, if respect and trust are absent the collaboration will more than likely fail.

CASE STUDY: AUTISM SOCIETY OF AMERICA REVISITED

Throughout its national system of chapters, the organization, by means of its grassroots volunteer base that touches thousands of people on a daily basis, works collaboratively on the local level with professionals, the government, and service agencies. Local chapters provide advocacy, education, and support to their local communities. The ASA chapters provide a wide array of services. Some are direct services such as residential programs, supportive and assistive employment, respite care, advocacy training, and direct support. Almost all work with the local professionals to assist with support for families, educating the community, and raising awareness and acceptance of autism.

On the national level, the ASA has been involved with virtually every major disability issue and piece of legislation impacting patients with autism since the mid-1960s. These include the Individuals with Disabilities Education Act (IDEA) of 1977, the Americans with Disabilities Act (ADA) of 1990, the Children's Health Act of 2000, the Combating Autism Act of 2006, and many others. These successes are primarily due to the collaborative efforts of the ASA working with multiple groups.

An example of professionals heeding the needs of a family-based organization was the publication of the landmark issue of the *Autism Advocate* in December 2006. This issue was devoted to publicizing the environmental factors that were thought to increase the incidence of autism and other developmental disabilities, and advocating for the advancement of treatments for autism. Since there were diverse and controversial opinions surrounding this subject, the ASA brought together the thought leaders in the field of autism to present their various perspectives in order to advance the science on how environmental factors contributed to the rise in autism and determine the next steps in order to advance treatment. What resulted was a wonderful exchange of ideas and consensus among all parties to leave the more controversial and divisive aspects of the subject to the side while focusing on what all could agree upon and what can be done in the short term.

A similar and equally successful collaborative effort was accomplished in 2008 when ASA joined with the Autism Research Institute and brought together 25 of the world's leading pediatric gastroenterologists to construct a consensus document addressing the issue of gastrointestinal disorders and autism. The importance of gastrointestinal issues to people with autism has been an area of some disagreement between health care professionals and family members and this consensus statement has made an appreciable difference in resolving these differences and is an excellent example of how professional/family collaborations can be of broad benefit. The work was a resounding success with the consensus document being published in the *Journal of Pediatrics*.

In general, the more successful ASA chapters are those that have strong and vibrant relationships with professionals in the community whom they actively engage in the leadership of the chapter.

CASE STUDY: FORMATION OF THE MIND INSTITUTE AT THE UNIVERSITY OF CALIFORNIA, DAVIS

The story of the founding and development of the MIND (Medical Investigation of Neurodevelopmental Disorders) Institute at the University of California, Davis (UCD) is one of great inspiration. It illustrates on a grand scale what professional and parent collaborations can do together. For a more comprehensive version of this story, see the Anders, Gardner, and Gardner (2003) chapter cited in the reference section.

Five families having children with autism were discouraged by the scant hope for successful treatment they received from the professionals who diagnosed each of their sons with autism. They were also confused and disappointed that each of the diverse professionals (child psychiatrists and psychologists, pediatric neurologists, developmental pediatricians) they took their children to see had differing approaches to their treatment and worked in isolation from each other. In addition, neither did educators nor other health professionals appear to communicate effectively with these professionals. Further, parents found that researchers into the causes of autism and other neurodevelopmental disorders and these clinicians seemed to work and think in separate domains. These parents dreamed of a place where all of the people interested in finding the cause, better treatments, and even cures for autism could work together.

The parents met with the leadership of the University of California Davis Medical Center (UCDMC) and each group began to develop an enthusiasm for what the great strength of their potential collaboration might produce. They met with the clinicians, educators, and researchers together in the same room and developed the beginning of a collaborative, integrative model.

An Executive Board was formed with equal numbers of members from the university and parent and community agencies, and they developed a partnership that held retreats, engaged in strategic planning, and the recruitment of new leadership. They developed a resource center and held educational events. They also developed a successful strategy for fund raising.

The challenges that the collaborative group described were: the differing styles of operating, the direction of the research and the clinical care, and the distribution of resources between missions and resources. Mutual respect and continual mutual education were both key to the success of this ongoing collaboration.

The result? Over 100 million dollars raised over 10 years from the State legislature, private philanthropists, and the UCDMC;

a new 100,000-square-foot building was built with clinics, interdisciplinary offices, and 30,000 square feet of wet lab space all designed to foster collaboration between health care professionals and researchers, educators, and families; the recruitment of an interdisciplinary team of researchers, clinicians, and educators; and the infrastructure to sustain this collaboration. This idea, started by parents and nourished through collaboration, grew through the collaborative recruitment of researchers and clinicians. Today, 250 people dedicated to understanding the causes and finding better treatments and cures for autism and neurodevelopmental disorders work together in this special building on the campus of the UCDMC. The MIND Institute has an annual budget of over 20 million dollars, mostly from Federal and foundation grants. Important progress has been made at the MIND Institute in the understanding and treatment of autism and other neurodevelopmental disorders and the program continues to grow through successful collaboration.

CASE STUDY: MY SON WITH AUTISM—AN ADVOCACY ODYSSEY AND MESSAGE FOR HEALTH PROFESSIONALS (BY LEE GROSSMAN)

At the time, the younger of my two sons was a sweet and good natured boy who was beginning to demonstrate language delays and seemed to be missing developmental milestones. The differences between him and his peers became more noticeable as he approached his third birthday. Despite the concerns of teachers and my sister, a psychologist, I maintained a wait-and-see attitude until my sister threatened to have my son taken away to get him the help he needed. This threat shocked me and spurred me into action. However, the opinions of pediatricians, child psychologists, developmental pediatricians, audiologists, child neurologists, psychiatrists, and educational experts varied greatly, ranging from, "There is nothing wrong," to "He is hopelessly retarded and needs to be institutionalized." Frustrated and confused, I spent several days in a local library attempting to find anything of relevance on the subject. Some books on autism that I found described in exact detail my son's symptoms and behaviors. The clarity of the descriptions was overwhelming to me and I broke down crying, completely convinced that my son had autism.

    I asked the professionals who had evaluated my son if they thought he had autism. Remember, this was the early 1990s. None would confirm the diagnosis, stating that my boy was too "friendly and caring" to have such a hopeless and profound diagnosis. At my sister's suggestion, desperate for help, I sought out a parent support group; fortunately, one had recently formed in our community.

I walked into a local chapter meeting of the ASA as a very frustrated, angry, and disgusted person. My attitude was that no one was experiencing what I was, that the group would be a waste of time, and that they would provide no assistance to me. I was unhappy to be there and clearly demonstrated it to the chapter members.

Within 10 minutes of walking through the door of the chapter meeting, I felt as though I had found a new family and a new home. The members of the chapter were very understanding of my predicament, had similar experiences, provided solutions, and were unselfish in their willingness to help and be a mentor to me. They provided valuable resources and referrals and attentively listened to my frustration and grief. They provided the personal touch and understanding that I had not yet found in the professional community, along with clarity and vision about the future. I then felt confident in moving forward. I met and developed a close relationship with Dr. Bernard Rimland and other professionals who were knowledgeable in the field, enabling me to obtain a correct diagnosis from one of the best autism centers in the nation.

I brought this new knowledge back to my local chapter. Over the next 3 years, I took on leadership positions in the chapter where we worked on successful State legislation to fund and maintain a technical assistance and resource center for autism, and establish model programs in autism. We held conferences and monthly educational meetings and support groups, and built the chapter into a respected, leading advocacy organization.

I cultivated relationships with innovative, respected experts and convinced them to share their expertise with their communities. I attended numerous autism conferences and visited model service agencies and medical groups around the country. My advocacy efforts extended from the local and State levels and on to Washington, DC. I also became active with the national ASA organization by communicating with them often and sharing ideas about local successes.

In 1995, realizing that the issues affecting families with autism would best be solved through a larger and more coordinated national effort, I ran for and was elected to the national ASA Board of Directors. In total, I served as the ASA's President and CEO for over 6 years and as Chair of the Board for an additional 4.

Today my son is a happy and healthy young adult with friends and interests that keep him involved and engaged in his community. I firmly believe that raising a child with a disability who will become a productive adult requires cooperation among agencies, professionals, other family members, and nonprofit groups.

I acknowledge the work that parents and advocates did before my son was diagnosed, the assistance of professionals who dedicate themselves to these families and individuals with disabilities, the ongoing devotion and passion that drive advocates, and the strength and remarkable courage borne each day by those having a disability or illness.

My experiences are not unique among advocates. The story of how my son was first diagnosed in the early 1990s is the similar experience many new families have today. I see the drive I have as an advocate in the eyes of most people who work in this field, and I hear the commensurate passion when they talk about the work they do on behalf of their loved ones. To work with so many advocates who sacrifice and devote so much to the betterment of others has truly humbled me. I hope my story provides a bit of insight about family members for those health professionals who are motivated to work with our organizations. We need your help.

REFLECTION QUESTIONS

1. What personal characteristics of a health professional do you think are most important to exhibit when approaching the leadership of a family or community organization with which to collaborate?
2. What barriers to collaboration have you experienced? Based on your reflection on these barriers and the content of this chapter, what would you do with a similar situation if you were to encounter them now?
3. If you and a representative from a family organization were to attend a meeting with a legislator, legislative aide, or leader of a government agency that you hope will support a shared policy or project, how would you suggest structuring the meeting when you discuss it prior to the actual appointment? Who should speak first? What points should each of you make? Who should have the most "air time"?

PRACTICE MAKES PERFECT

1. Ask several family members of patients in your practice if they belong or have belonged to a family organization for the disorder their family member has. Why do they attend or why did they stop going? What did they find useful about attending? What were their disappointments? Did professionals attend? If so, what was useful in their attendance? Who were effective leaders in the organization?

2. Do an online search to locate a family or community-based organization focused on an advocacy issue of importance to you. Who is listed online for you to contact? How would you initially reach out?
3. Prepare a draft presentation that you might offer to give at a family or community organization or for a conference attended by professionals and family members. Does it contain enough accessible "science" for the intended audience? Do you have enough "vignettes" to engage your audience? Have you discussed some aspects that illustrate "family choice"? Have you left adequate but not too much time for discussion?

REFERENCES

Anders, T. F., Gardner, C. R., & Gardner, S. E. (2003). Professional-parent collaboration. In S. Ozonoff, S. Rogers, & R. L. Hendren (Eds.), *Autism spectrum disorders: A research review for practitioners* (pp. 227–238). Washington, DC: American Psychiatric Publishing, Inc.

Hoagwood, K. E., Cavaleri, M. A., Serene, O. S., Burns, B. J., Slaton, E., Gruttadaro, D., & Hughes, R. (2010). Family support in children's mental health: A review and synthesis. *Clinical Child and Family Psychology Review, 13*(1), 1–45.

Ochoa, E. R., Jr., & Nash, C. (2009). Community engagement and its impact on child health disparities: Building blocks, examples, and resources. *Pediatrics, 124*(Suppl. 3), S237–S245.

10

Finding Funds

TRACY MILLS

There is partnership in philanthropy. We need grantees. We are only an enabler of good work.—Roxanne Ford,
W.M. Keck Foundation (Geever, 2004)

This chapter covers the nuts and bolts of fundraising to support your advocacy mission. Contrary to intuition, fundraising at its core is not about raising money. Fundraising is about having a vision—for a research project, a clinic, a better way of treating patients, an innovation in the field, a new hospital, a new opportunity—and sharing this vision with like-minded individuals who want to join you in seeing it become a reality. Most philanthropists will explain that the largest gifts they make are just as meaningful to them as they are to the organizations that receive the support. Health care professionals who can identify grateful patients and families committed to preventing and curing diseases and involve them in meaningful ways with the organization will be well-positioned to inspire this type of philanthropy. The word *philanthropy* roughly translates to "love of man," reminding you that when you articulate your mission with concrete uses for the donor's funding it must be tied to a clear benefit for people and society.

FUNDING SOURCES

Private support has become increasingly important in health care settings. As Federal and State funding continues to decline and insurance reimbursements become more restricted, health care professionals are turning to private support to fill gaps in clinical services and launch new research projects. In 2009, of the $303.75 billion in U.S. national giving, health care organizations accounted for $22.46 billion, education for $40.01 billion, and giving to public and human services was another $49.85 billion (Figure 10.1; Giving USA Foundation, 2010).

The majority of national giving comes from individuals, who give more than all other groups combined. In 2009, approximately 83% of all private philanthropy in the United States was given by individuals, foundations accounted for 13%, and corporations made up the final 4% of giving (Figure 10.2; Giving USA Foundation, 2010). Of the $38.44 billion in foundation grants, it is estimated that $15.41 billion came from family foundations. It seems clear that health care professionals with limited time and resources should focus their energy on searching for individual partners to support their projects. Patients and families are a good match for fundraising opportunities because of their deep and personal understanding of the impact of the diseases that these health care professionals are fighting.

These three groups—individuals, corporations, and foundations—have different motivations for investing in philanthropy and different expectations in return. Individuals are motivated to make gifts that support ideas, causes, and people. In health care, they give because they want to thank a professional who helped them or their family, because they want to help others, or because they want to advance the field of science in a disease area. Individuals do not expect anything in return for their gifts but they appreciate recognition and updates from the people they are supporting.

Contrast this with foundations, whose giving is analogous to an outsourcing relationship with a philanthropic partner. Established foundations have clearly defined priorities and strategies for how they want to invest their funding (Caruso, 2008). Often they have measured goals they hope to achieve. However, what foundations lack is the infrastructure to

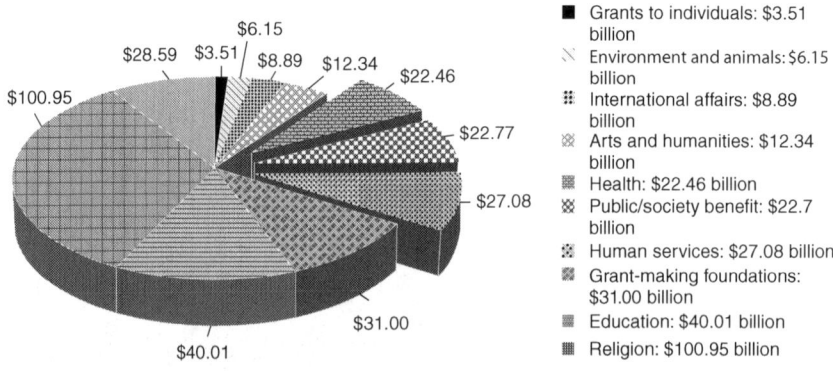

FIGURE 10.1
National Giving by Type of Recipient Organization, 2009: $303.75 Billion

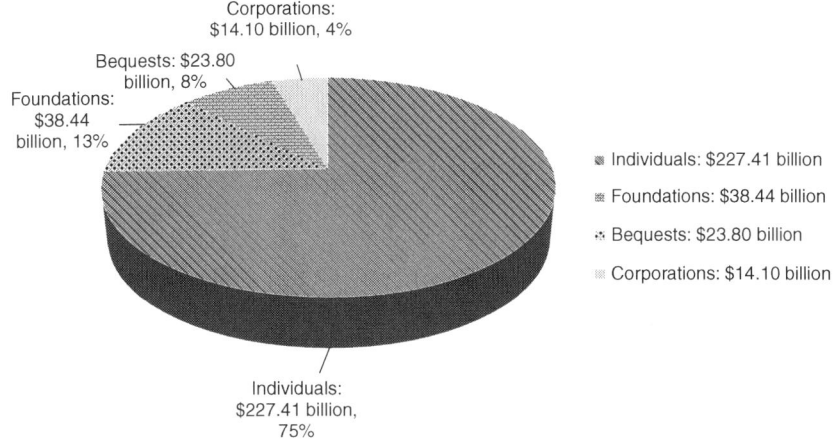

FIGURE 10.2
National Giving by Source of Contributions, 2009: $303.75 Billion

accomplish their priorities independently. They may have a desire to cure diabetes, but they do not have the doctors, nurses, research labs, clinics, and patients to work toward this goal. Foundations will enter into an outsourcing relationship with the partner that is best suited to achieve their mission in the way they envision it. When a medical program and a foundation are aligned in mission, methodology, and strategy, there is the greatest opportunity for health care professionals to receive grant funding. In return for this funding, foundations expect well-defined plans, accountability, and regular reporting.

Corporations make investments in their community, workforce, and reputation. Corporate partners seek philanthropic investments that add value back to the corporation (Mills, 2008). They will support training programs that advance their workforce (Kraus, 1998), social services that enhance the communities where they have offices or where their customers live, and public events where they will be recognized for their contribution. For example, a corporation may invest in malaria prevention in a country where it has its manufacturing base or it may support a charity event for cancer research in a community where it has local offices (Callahan, 2008). When working with corporate partners, it is essential to define what is in it for them. In return for funding, corporations expect mutually beneficial plans, accountability, and regular reporting.

Fundraising Roles and Responsibilities

Health care professionals can take comfort in the fact that although fundraising can be challenging, you should not have to do it alone. Many health care professionals engaged in advocacy work are affiliated with major institutions or agencies that have a development or advancement office with a staff of professional fundraisers who can support your efforts to find private funding. A sophisticated development infrastructure will have annual giving fundraisers, major giving fundraisers, planned giving officers, corporate and foundation relations officers, prospect research, alumni services, event planning, development communications, gift and endowment accounting, and a formal 501(c)(3) foundation. However, even if your office has only a director of development, she can still be your best partner in fundraising.

The director of development is responsible for raising major gifts for your institution. She serves as a bridge between health care professionals and development resources. She helps you identify potential major donors among your grateful patients and provides research on the prospect's background and wealth indicators. The director of development helps design strategies for cultivating and soliciting prospects at the most appropriate amount, plans cultivation and solicitation meetings, and prepares written materials. The development office creates binding legal documents for accepting gifts and pledges, and provides services for the prompt acknowledgment of gifts. Finally, the director of development ensures donors' gifts are being properly stewarded and coordinates the donor's relationship with the entire institution.

The director of development guides and assists the health care provider in fundraising, but the primary relationship resides with the donor and the health care provider. The health care professional sets the mission for the program, project, or department and articulates the goals and needs. The director of development looks to health care professionals to identify grateful patients or friends of the institution who are good fundraising prospects. Health care professionals are expected to participate in donor cultivation and solicitation and to convey the value and results of philanthropic support. Health care professionals also bring prestige to the institution and provide credibility and expertise. At times health care professionals struggle with the ethics of asking their patients to philanthropically support their work. It is helpful to remember that philanthropy is not about asking your patients to do something they are hesitant or reluctant to do or asking for a personal favor. Fundraising is about presenting your vision for the future and giving the patients the opportunity to invest in something that has personal meaning to them. It should always be made clear to the patient that quality care is given to all patients regardless of their interest or willingness to make a gift. Development directors are a useful bridge and can help to professionalize the philanthropic relationship between the donor and the institution.

Development directors are often asked to help with brochures, annual appeal letters, and development events. Although these activities are useful for outreach, the vast majority of philanthropy comes from

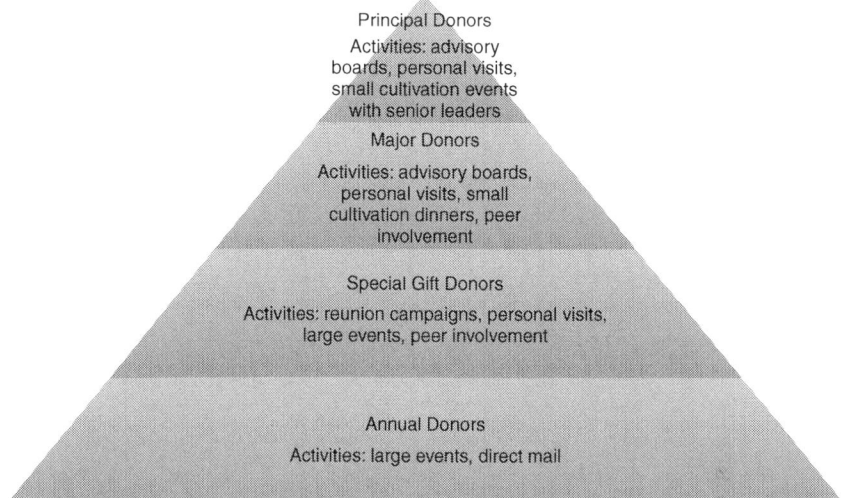

FIGURE 10.3
Donor Pyramid by Level and Activities.

"major gifts" to the institution. These gifts, generally $100,000 and above, are the result of high-touch, personal, face-to-face solicitations rather than letters and galas. Major gifts from the top donors can account for 80%–90% of the fundraising for an institution. In contrast, low-touch activities such as letters and events create a larger volume of gifts and are useful in acquiring new donors and beginning to build relationships, but they generally bring in a much smaller percentage of total giving.

FUNDRAISING FROM INDIVIDUALS

Development is about fostering relationships with donors and inspiring them with the vision of what you can achieve together. Each individual has his or her own reasons, but there are general themes around what motivates donors to give.

The reasons donors give to worthy causes (Leonhardt, 2008):
- To invest in a cause that has personal meaning to them.
- To thank or honor an individual who has helped them.
- To ensure the future.
- To honor the past.
- To help others less fortunate.
- To continue a family tradition of giving.
- To have a personal impact.
- To leave a legacy.
- To receive recognition among their peers (BBC News, 2008).
- To receive tax benefits.

Donors give to worthy causes:
- When they are involved in the organization or cause.
- When they feel an emotional connection.
- When someone they respect asks them to give.
- When they support the mission.
- When they wish to honor someone.
- When they feel the organization is well-managed and effective.
- When they understand how the funding will be used.
- When the organization listens to their interests and matches their priorities.
- Most importantly, when they are asked.

Donors choose not to give or stop giving to a cause (Colorado Nonprofit Association, 2008):
- When the project is not a good match for their interests or priorities.
- When the timing is not right personally or financially.
- When they no longer feel connected to the organization.
- When they decide other causes are more worthy of their support.
- When they have not been properly thanked for prior giving.
- When they feel they are solicited too often.

The common thread that underlies giving by individuals is that they have developed a personal connection to the cause or the person asking for support. Since the largest gifts are the result of these long-term relationships, health care professionals will be advised to move fundraising prospects through a series of stages that will develop the relationships

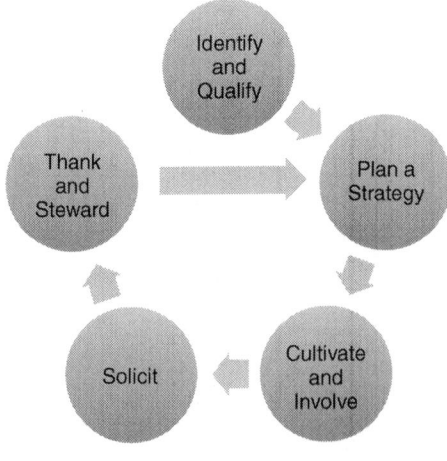

FIGURE 10.4
Fundraising Cycle.

over time. The development lifecycle (Rosso, 1991a) moves through the process of identifying potential donors, determining the best strategy, cultivating and involving prospects, preparing for and making the solicitation, and thanking and stewarding the gift.

Identify and Qualify

Health care professionals are the frontline in terms of identifying prospective donors among patients and their families. A large percentage of fundraising in health care comes from grateful patients who will self-identify if health care professionals are listening for cues that they want to get more involved.

Signs that the patient is a potential prospect for supporting the cause for which you are advocating:

- They express an interest in learning more about your work.
- They take interest in advancing scientific discovery or helping other families.
- They express gratitude to you and a desire to give back.
- They seek out your expertise and acknowledge situations where you have gone above and beyond the call of duty.
- They talk about their other philanthropy.

Identification is only the first step in the process, however. Once you have identified a prospect, you then need to qualify this interest and begin engaging the person. This is a time for you to describe your vision and to learn more about the individuals priorities and values. Here you will talk about what inspires you in your job, why you chose the work you do, and what you see in the future. You will share your goals and dreams with the prospects and ask for their advice. You will tell them about the people in your department and the innovative research or clinical programs taking place at your institution. You will describe the needs of the institution and what you would be able to accomplish with more resources. This is also the time where you want to learn more about the prospects and their motivations to get involved. Find out why they have an interest in your area of specialty, what it means to them, and what they would like to see in the future. Ask if they are involved with other nonprofit organizations and what they find meaningful in that work.

There are many factors that influence a donor's willingness to make a gift to an organization. Some donors make their philanthropic decisions in partnership with their spouses or children. Others look for opportunities to be involved with organizations that are connected to their friends or business associates. Personal finances and the current economic environment

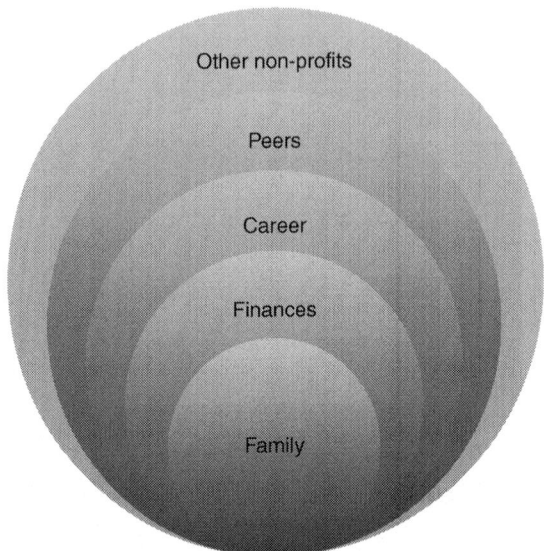

FIGURE 10.5
Factors influencing philanthropic decisions.

clearly can affect a donor's ability to make a gift. Similarly a busy career and family life can have an impact. Donors who are entering retirement may be looking for a place to impart their skills and wisdom. Older donors may begin to think about their legacy and impact on the next generation. Donors involved with other non-profits may have prior philanthropic commitments and multi-year pledges. Development officers can conduct research to determine a donor's financial assets such as stock holdings, public salary information, and real estate (Rosso, 1991b). Because there are so many elements that can influence the likelihood and ideal timing of a solicitation, it is important to gather as much information as you can when you qualify a donor (Campbell & Company Research Fellow, 2006).

Plan a Strategy

Planning a solicitation strategy is one of the most important components in a successful solicitation. Too often fundraising falls short when medical professionals do not think about how to properly approach the donor and the discussion of philanthropy. The following are ten elements to consider when planning a strategy:

1. Capacity—What is the prospect's financial ability to make a gift?
2. Interest—What are the prospect's personal and philanthropic interests?

3. Inclination—How inclined is the prospect to make a gift to the program?
4. Relationships—Who is the prospect most connected to in the organization?
5. Other philanthropic priorities—Does this organization rank high on the donor's list of charities?
6. Motivation—What would motivate the prospect to make a gift? Who is the right person to make the solicitation?
7. Messaging—What reasons are most compelling to the donor (helping others, helping find a cure, etc.)? What aspect of the program would they be most interested in supporting (endowed chairs, fellowships, research funds, clinical support)?
8. Assets—Given the donor's personal situation, will they likely make a gift of cash, securities, or real estate or will it be an estate gift such as a bequest or gift annuity?
9. Amount—What is the appropriate gift amount given the purpose?
10. Timing—Given their financial commitments and personal interest, when is the right time to ask for the gift? Will the gift be made today or over time?

Cultivate and Involve

In fundraising, cultivation is the process of nurturing and growing the relationship with the prospective donor. For health care professionals, this process begins as soon as you interact with your patients in the health care setting. The way you treat your patients, the care that you provide for them, the time you take answering their questions, and your genuine concern for their health and well-being are all part of the cultivation process. These are actions you take regardless of a patient's ability to make a donation, and skilled health care professionals will have many grateful patients, some who will be donors and others who will express their gratitude in different ways.

When you have identified a grateful patient that you believe has the capacity and inclination to make a gift to your program, you can begin to cultivate the patient outside of the health care setting. Cultivation can take multiple forms: inviting the patient to a tour of your lab or a new facility, taking him to lunch or visiting him at home, inviting her to research presentations or seminars, or introducing him to key colleagues. The cultivation process is an opportunity to educate the prospect about the strengths of the department and the compelling aspects of your work. As you meet with prospects, it is important to think carefully and creatively about their personal motivations and goals and involve them in ways that would be most meaningful to them. When you created your strategy, you developed a plan for what you think they would most like to support. Now is the time to demonstrate to the prospect the qualities and benefits of your work through interactions with colleagues, students, and others involved in the program.

Cultivation of a prospect can take months and even years. As the relationship grows over time, so will the commitment and the amount of the gift. As time passes, however, it is important to keep the prospect engaged. Grateful patients can have life-changing experiences within hospital walls, yet the willingness of a patient to give is highest within 3 months of receiving care (WealthEngine, 2010) and declines dramatically over time after the care has ceased. It is critical to engage these patients before they become distanced from the organization and the experience.

CASE STUDY: CULTIVATING A RELATIONSHIP

Julie's son was seen at a specialty clinic for a severe and debilitating illness. The clinic conducted a series of tests and gave her a diagnosis that finally answered her many questions about what was affecting her son. Although the clinic was not equipped to treat her son, they were able to refer him to another facility that could give him the care he needed. Julie was extremely grateful to the clinic's director, Dr. A, both for the relief of finally having a diagnosis, but also for Dr. A's optimism that her son might be able to recover from his illness. Julie sent a note to Dr. A, thanking her for her help, encouragement, and care. A few weeks later, Dr. A noticed Julie's name in a publication about philanthropy at her institution. As it turned out, Julie was the executive director of her family's foundation and had been working on a fundraising project for another program.

Dr. A responded to Julie's note and the two began a conversation about the clinic and its current work. Over time, Julie and Dr. A agreed that if the clinic had the ability to treat a greater percentage of the patients they were diagnosing, it would offer more consistency and ease of care for the families. Julie asked Dr. A to send her a proposal to expand the services of the clinic. Through this initial gift and during the course of subsequent interactions, Julie's connection grew from someone who had experience with the clinic and an understanding of the cause, to someone who felt a sense of ownership and involvement with the clinic.

As with many private foundations, Julie's family foundation was inclined to support programs that would not solely rely on their support and could raise matching funding. Therefore, in order to submit a second and larger proposal to the foundation, Dr. A needed to fundraise from other prospective donors. Since she was committed to the success of the program, Julie offered to meet with donors to the clinic to encourage them to match the funds of her family's foundation. Julie was the ideal volunteer–fundraiser because she understood personally what made the clinic so important and she was willing to speak about her son's experience and reflect for others on the impact of her philanthropy. One of these early meetings involved another foundation also interested in leveraging its grants through matching funds. Julie told the story of how the clinic had helped her son and gave an inspiring pitch for why the two foundations should work together to help other families. Because of Julie's encouragement and as a direct result of a meeting between these two foundations, both agreed to make a $250,000 pledge, each gift matching the other.

As you cultivate a donor, both before and after the gift, at each stage you are bringing them closer to the organization. Grateful patients start with awareness of the organization, which grows into interest and experience as they become more connected. Ideally, you want your prospects to move beyond experience and feel a sense of ownership of the organization. By engaging them as volunteers, asking for their advice, and asking them to reach out to others, you deepen their commitment. In return, it is your responsibility to ensure the donor feels valued by and is valuable to the organization.

CASE STUDY: THE IMPORTANCE OF CONNECTIONS

Martha was an experienced philanthropist involved with many organizations. Years before, her son was in a severe car accident and suffered from a traumatic brain injury that would plague him for the rest of his life. The doctors thought he wouldn't graduate from high school, but he recently received his second advanced degree from a major university. Martha's son was able to overcome many obstacles, but his brain injury still affected his personal and working relationships. Because of her interest, Martha was introduced by a mutual friend to a mental health clinic that is working with veterans returning home from war. Many of these veterans suffered from similar traumatic brain injury but the stigma of receiving mental health care kept them from seeking help and services. Since Martha understood on a personal level the difficulties faced by these veterans and the need for support, she started to become involved in the clinic and introduced the clinic's director to other non-profits' leaders working with veterans. These connections resulted in the launch of a new college program teaching veterans how to use the skills and strengths they learned in the military and how to manage post-traumatic stress and traumatic brain injury.

Since the clinic was able to capitalize on Martha's connections with local colleges and other non-profits, Martha next hosted a reception at her house to raise awareness about the issues facing veterans. She invited other friends she thought would have a connection to the cause and the clinic invited current donors to help carry the message of the need for support. The evening included a presentation where people involved with the clinic—veterans, faculty members, military leaders—told stories that described their experience and showed the need for the program and the benefits to the community. One of Martha's friends grew up in a military family and felt an instant connection to the cause and is now an active member of the clinic's advisory board. The evening resulted in three new five-figure gifts for the clinic, including one from Martha.

Solicit

When you have determined the timing is right to ask for a gift, keep in mind that each individual solicitation will be different and should be tailored to the individual. Some prospects will prefer a formal proposal not unlike one that you would submit to a foundation. With other donors you may begin with a dialogue and formalize the conversation with a gift agreement. In any case, the prospect should not be surprised by the request (Dahnert, 1998). When you schedule the appointment, you should be upfront that you plan to discuss the needs of the program and how they can help support your mission. The decision to make a large gift takes time and careful reflection, so it is in your best interest to give the prospect a chance to prepare in advance for the conversation.

The "ask" should come from the person who has the closest relationship to the donor and can speak to the needs of the program. It is also important that the request come from a person in a position of authority—often a senior leader in the organization, the health care professional who cared for the patient, or a volunteer peer who has made his or her own commitment to the cause. Prospects will want to know that this project is a priority for the organization, and key leaders can demonstrate the project's importance.

The gift discussion should be well planned and should reflect the values and priorities of interest to the donor. During the qualification and cultivation stages, you learn from the donors about the factors that influence their philanthropy—what motivates them to give, who should be included in the gift discussion, and why they are interested in your cause. You carefully listen for cues and incorporate what you hear into the case for support. Philanthropy is fundamentally about fulfilling the donor's desire to make a positive change in an area of personal importance. This is not a time to discuss the dire circumstances or negative consequences of the lack of funding. You will be successful if you can inspire the prospect to make a gift but you will not be able to depress them into making one! If a solicitation goes well, the donor will walk away as excited to make the gift as you are to receive it.

Asking for a gift can be stressful and so rehearsing in advance how you will approach the discussion can help alleviate concerns and refine your messaging. Once you have stated your case for support and made the "ask," you need to stop talking and give the donor the chance to respond. If the donor does not immediately reply, give them a minute to reflect and gather their thoughts. An anxious solicitor will sometimes keep talking straight through the "ask" and walk away from the meeting unsure about the donor's reaction. This is an important time to hear from the donors about why they are excited to support the cause, any concerns they have, or why they cannot support the cause at this time. This is a critical moment to gather information that will inform your next steps and future solicitations.

CASE STUDY: THE IMPORTANCE OF FOCUSING ON THE DONOR

Carol is a notably wealthy individual. Early in her career, she volunteered at a public hospital and met a faculty member there working on internet-based health care interventions. Over the next few years, they worked together on a few collaborative projects and Carol helped connect Dr. B with industry contacts to promote his work. They had several conversations about philanthropy and Carol suggested that she had an interest in supporting two of the projects that Dr. B was currently undertaking. Dr. B eventually submitted a six-figure proposal to Carol, which she did not respond to for some time. When Carol received word through a mutual friend that Dr. B's project was in jeopardy, she sent Dr. B $100,000, half of the amount he had originally asked for in the proposal.

Another year passed and Carol and Dr. B continued to have contact through a joint collaboration. Dr. B invited Carol to meet again to discuss her philanthropic support of his program. Carol suggested that she was very busy but Dr. B should send her another proposal. Dr. B consulted with the development officer and they decided that the proposal should set a bold vision for the future of the program and include support that would be sustaining over several years. The hope was that if Carol was not willing to fund the full proposal, she would be inspired by the vision and would help connect Dr. B with other individuals with an interest in this work. The proposal Dr. B sent was for $5 million to establish a Center that would support Dr. B's work over the next 5 years, allowing the program to complete several key projects of interest to Carol.

After numerous attempts, Carol still has not responded to the proposal sent more than a year ago. In retrospect some of the factors that made this solicitation unsuccessful seem clear, but at the time they were encouraged by her request for a proposal and swept up by her capacity to make a large gift. Three key elements were missing from the solicitation: (a) There was not enough of a dialogue with Carol to find out what level of proposal she was most comfortable in considering. They were more concerned with what level of gift she was capable of making rather than assessing her commitment to the program. (b) They let the needs of the program dictate the amount rather than the donor's willingness to give. (c) They did not properly prepare her for the size of the proposal and take cues from her past philanthropy and the fact that she only funded half of the previous proposal at $100,000.

If a prospect refuses to fund a proposal it does not mean you have failed. "No" is not the same as "never." Perhaps it is an issue of timing and the current economic climate. In a declining economy, donors may not feel as confident in their personal wealth and may not be in a position to donate their assets. Tax incentives that come with making charitable contributions may not be as relevant when donors are experiencing financial losses. Or perhaps the issue is that the donor has not been sold enough on the cause. Rather than abandon the relationship, it is a good time to return to the cultivation stage and reassess your strategy. Rejections are common in fundraising but each one can be a valuable learning process.

Thank and Steward

Once a gift or pledge has been committed, you need to thank the donor and begin to cultivate her for the next gift. You do this by being a good steward of the gift, by using the funds appropriately, and by providing reports and updates on what her generosity has allowed you to accomplish. Donors rarely begin a philanthropic relationship with the largest gift they are capable of making. More often they will begin the relationship slowly and the initial contribution will help them decide if they want to continue to support the program. New donors are introduced to an organization by current donors when positive relationships are maintained and gifts have been well stewarded.

Maintaining donor relationships requires forethought, and a stewardship plan will help you continue to reach out and connect with the donor throughout the year. Different people will find different activities meaningful and so the best stewardship plans are tailored to the individual donor. Most donors appreciate receiving written reports about the impact their gift made to the program and helping other patients. Some donors will want high visibility and public recognition of their gift through naming opportunities, articles in institutional publications, and ceremonies. Others will appreciate small dinners where they are able to meet the students or families they support or interact with notable health care leaders at the institution.

Stewardship is also about making donors feel needed and important. You do this by asking for their advice and including them in your plans and programs. You ask them to give again, to consider giving more, and to invite others to give. When they are asked to give, it is by someone who is important in the organization and who genuinely feels excited about the program and its accomplishments. Well-stewarded donors feel like they can share with others the importance of making a gift to the organization because you have shown them the results.

CASE STUDY: REMEMBER TO CONTINUE COMMUNICATING WITH DONORS

A few years back, George, grateful for the care he received at his local medical center, endowed a faculty Chair in a specialty area of intellectual interest to him. It was a unique subject area for the hospital and it took the organization several years to fill the position. George grew increasingly frustrated by the amount of time that had lapsed with the position unfilled and he felt his gift was not valued by the organization. When the Chair holder finally arrived, the department set out to mend these ties with George. The development officer arranged a small dinner with George, his daughter, the new faculty member, the department chair, and the faculty member who originally inspired George to make the gift. At the dinner it was clear that George was excited to meet his new chair holder, Dr. C. He was very interested in her research and was beginning to feel connected to the organization again.

When a reception was planned to welcome Dr. C to the hospital, George was invited to attend and he was presented with an award for his dedication to the organization. Dr. C and George continued to periodically meet for lunch to discuss her work and his interests in the subject area. As time passed, George, excited by Dr. C's research, began to discuss other financial resources he could provide to help expand her work. Instead of making a list of ways George could support her, Dr. C continually thanked George for his generosity and they agreed that together they would think about a vision for the future of the program. George is now discussing with Dr. C the idea of building a center to support Dr. C's specialty area and Dr. C is carefully crafting a plan for what resources would be needed to make the center successful. George suggested that in a year they would meet for dinner again, this time at George's house, to celebrate how far the program has come since that first evening together.

VOLUNTEERS

Volunteers are often our best sources of philanthropy. Of course not all volunteers have the capacity to make a large donation, but for those who do, the experience of volunteering helps connect them with the organization and its mission and gives them a sense of ownership and pride. Engaging grateful patients as volunteers has advantages: Many health care professionals find it more comfortable to ask for guidance, advice, and volunteer of assistance than for money. Involving a potential donor as a volunteer enables you to discuss with that person your vision for the future and the financial resources necessary to achieve these goals before initiating a conversation about a gift.

One of the ways that fundraisers involve volunteers is through advisory boards or committees (DiConsiglio, 2011). An advisory council is generally made up of people interested in supporting your cause and gives you a sounding board for your fundraising messages. It is also a useful way to connect a group of potential donors and offers structured communication and cultivation in the form of regular committee meetings. These types of advisory councils are merely consultative and have no governing power or budget authority over the organization, but members should know that they are being asked to serve because they have strengths and skills that are useful. It is important that volunteers know what you are asking of them and that you use their time wisely. Offering a job description for advisory council members is a useful starting point to make sure that organizational expectations are matched by the volunteer.

Advisory councils serve an important role in public relations as well as providing an outside perspective on your programs and work. Advisory council members serve as a role model for others and as a public ambassador for the organization. It is often expected that they will make a personal contribution to the organization and help connect the organization with other individuals interested in the cause. You want them to be informed about the organization—its culture, mission, and needs—and you should tell them stories that describe the impact of the organization so that they can remember and repeat these stories when fundraising on your behalf.

In return for their service, volunteers want to feel recognized by the organization—they want to be invited to special activities and lectures, introduced to inspiring doctors, listened to when they give advice or guidance, and acknowledged for their efforts.

CASE STUDY: KEEPING DONORS INVOLVED WITH YOUR CAUSE

Marc Benioff, the founder of SalesForce.com, is a young billionaire entrepreneur who has ingrained corporate giving into his company's mission (Duxbury, 2011). At 45, Marc had already given over $20 million to a number of different charitable causes but this philanthropy had always left him wanting more (Barret, 2010). Marc had supported orphanages, schools, and monasteries with mixed result and he felt that he wanted to make a gift and see that it was having an impact (Guth, 2011). Marc's wife Lynne served on the Advisory Board of the University of California, San Francisco, and after his daughter was born at the hospital, they endowed four faculty Chairs at UCSF. When asked to make a gift to the campaign for the University's new hospital and research center, Marc agreed to an anonymous $20 million gift and to volunteer to help bring in new support.

Marc partnered with the hospital's CEO, Mark Laret, and the two started meeting with other billionaires to convince them that the hospital was a good investment. Through the process of convincing others, Marc began to convince himself. He began researching medical philanthropy and asking the advice of others who had funded hospitals. They repeatedly told him that medical philanthropy was the best thing they had ever done. Marc decided the time was right to fully commit to the hospital and make a legacy gift of $100 million. He also vowed to give exclusively to the hospital over the next 10 years. Marc's remarkable gift has only deepened his commitment to helping the hospital succeed, and he continues to serve as a tireless advocate and fundraiser for its mission.

FINAL POINTS TO REMEMBER ABOUT PRIVATE DONORS

If you focus on building meaningful and respectful relationships with donors, and clearly communicate the needs and impact of your advocacy, you will be successful in raising support. The following rules will help guide your attempts and keep things in perspective.

1. **It is not all about you.** Philanthropy is about fulfilling a donor's desire to have a positive impact on the world. Rather than helping you meet your goals, it is about finding a meaningful project that helps them realize their dreams (Rosso, 1991c).
2. **It is not all about donors.** Donors will sometimes have their own vision for your program. Make sure the project they want to fund is useful to you and the institution. If it is not, it is more respectful to discuss the issues and come to a mutual plan than to agree to something that is not a good fit. You need to make sure that the donor's expectations are aligned with what is reasonable and realistic for the organization.
3. **It takes time.** On average, it takes at least five substantive interactions with a donor before they will be willing to make a significant gift. However, the cultivation process begins with the health care provider and the patient in the clinical setting. Be sure you have properly established the relationship and prepared the prospect before you make the solicitation. Expect that the donor may want to start with a smaller gift and evaluate your ability to spend the funds wisely.
4. **It is all about you.** Donors will give to the causes and people they feel most passionately about. The relationship you have with the donors, the way you treat them, and the way you approach their philanthropy are of critical importance. There are numerous organizations worthy of a donor's support but the donor is most likely to give to the cause where they have developed the closest relationship and have been engaged and involved.
5. **Stay positive.** Philanthropy is about making positive change. Focusing on averting disaster, negative consequences, and dire circumstances will not inspire someone to make a gift. You can describe the negative elements you are facing, but it is important to keep the message focused on how the gift will help people rather than keep people from harm.
6. **Tell the external story rather than the internal story.** Rather than telling the donors why the funding is important to you, explain why it is important to them. Instead of describing the needs of the clinic, describe the needs of the patients you serve. Likewise, rather than focusing on the impact the gift will have on your program, focus on the impact the program will have on others.
7. **Be prepared and know your case.** When meeting with the donor make sure you understand the program's strengths and weaknesses. Partner with others if they are more qualified to describe the program and its impact.

8. **Show results.** Donors want to see and meet the people they have helped. Activities where you can share with the donor the results of their gift will lead to a deeper commitment and future philanthropy.
9. **There is partnership in philanthropy.** Gifts are not merely transactions; they are partnerships. Each partner brings an important resource to the project and each should be listened to and respected for what he or she contributes.
10. **You cannot thank a donor too much.** Stewardship is the most important element in philanthropy and leads to inspired donors who will continue to give back over years to come. A gift should be as rewarding to the donor who gives it as it is to the provider who receives it.

FOUNDATIONS AND CORPORATIONS

Although corporate and foundation philanthropy is not as significant as giving from individuals, in 2009 it still accounted for $52.54 billion of private support and can be a worthwhile source of funding for health care programs. As discussed earlier, foundations and corporations differ in their funding motivations and are more likely to enter into business-like transactions rather than emotion-driven philanthropy. Here your solicitation will likely be a formal proposal with quantifiable outcomes and objectives. A benefit to corporate and foundation fundraising is the transparency of information about the funder's priorities, amount of available funding, and grant-making process. With individuals, you have to ask artful and strategic questions to assess the donor's interests, priorities, and resources. For foundations and corporations, much of this information is publically available on their websites and in their tax documents.

Since so much information is readily available about foundations and corporations, research is an integral component of this form of fundraising. There are many non-profit websites available to help you create lists of foundations and corporations that are interested in funding your cause. Research can also help you determine a funder's giving capacity and whether they are likely to fund the program in the amount you need. Although many foundations have websites describing their grant-making process, you should also look at their IRS 990-PF tax documents to see the projects and amounts of the grants they are funding. The 990-PFs are the tax documents filed by private foundations in the United States (The Foundation Center, 2011) and are publically available at nonprofit sites such as GuideStar (guidestar.org) and The Foundation Center (foundationcenter.org). They detail the contact information for the foundation, the amount of gifts the foundation received, as well as the foundation's revenue, assets, and expenses. They also detail the grants paid with the amounts, and list the officers, directors, trustees, and key employees. Knowing the key decision makers at a foundation can prove useful in leveraging contacts and finding out if you have any personal connections.

Once you have discovered a foundation or corporation that matches your project, you will likely begin with a letter of inquiry or initial phone call. A letter of inquiry is an abbreviated version of a full proposal and should describe a singular project with a specific amount over a defined period of time. A letter of inquiry allows the foundation to assess whether the project is a good match and saves you the time of writing (and them of reviewing) a full proposal if the project is not going to be funded. The letter of inquiry should follow the same framework as the full proposal but will only be one to three pages. Generally a letter of inquiry and a full proposal will include: a summary section, a statement of need, the project description, proposed outcomes, your credentials and ability to carry out the project, an evaluation plan, budget, and closing section.

Some key considerations to remember when writing a letter of inquiry or a proposal to a foundation or corporation are:

1. **Tailor your strengths to their priorities.** Because information about a foundation's philanthropic priorities is widely available, you should explicitly explain how your project reflects these interests. In an outsourcing or investing relationship, a project that does not reflect the foundation or corporation's goals is not likely to be funded. With corporate proposals you want to clearly describe the benefit of the project to the corporation or how they will be recognized for their support (Cornforth, 1999).
2. **Summarize your case early in the proposal.** In the first paragraph state: who you are, your objective, the impact their grant will have, and the amount you are asking them to fund. You want the reviewer to know the answers to these four questions and make it easy for them to remember your case for support.
3. **Show rather than tell** (Jarrell, 2005). Funders review a number of proposals and you want yours to instantly register with the reviewer. The reviewer should not have to work to understand what you are trying to do and how you will accomplish your goals. Even though you are applying to a foundation or a corporation, there is still a person on the other end reading your application among a great big stack of others. No matter what the project is, an anecdote, illustration, quotation, or example will help make the abstract a reality. A good example in a proposal reflects the impact your project has on the community through the experience of an individual.

4. **Be clear and concise** (King, 1989). A funder may or may not be experienced in your area of specialty. Either way, it is your responsibility to make the proposal understandable and accessible. Avoiding technical terms and institutional jargon will help the reader understand your project.
5. **Demonstrate the positive impact.** Funders want to make impactful change in the world rather than avert disaster. Any negative statement can be rewritten into a positive statement that describes the benefits of philanthropy. For example, rather than focusing on the number of deaths related to a particular disease, describe what it is like for a person to regain their life. Instead of painting a picture of the trauma of illness on a child, focus on the promise that a young healthy life holds. You want to leave the reader feeling hopeful for the future rather than saddened by the current state of the world.
6. **Be confident but do not overstate your case.** It is important to reference your credentials and describe why you are ideally suited to carry out this project. Your proposal should portray the excellence of your program but should also support any claims you make with facts. It is tempting to make grand statements about your program, but if they are questionable, these may cost you your credibility.
7. **Make it manageable and measurable.** Foundations and corporations are increasingly looking for innovative and impactful projects with well-thought-out evaluation plans. Foundations hold themselves and their program officers accountable for the outcomes and results of the projects they fund, and they want to make sure their grant-making dollars are put to the best use.
8. **Open and close with a clear call to action.** People use passive language and bury the funding request in proposals because they feel guilty asking for money. Your proposal should begin with an active statement about the project and what you are asking from the foundation or corporation. Likewise, you should close the proposal with a reiteration of the request and detail of the next steps in the process.

A well-crafted letter of inquiry for a worthwhile project will hopefully result in a request for a full proposal, a site visit, or perhaps even a grant agreement. If you are awarded the grant, be sure to note the reporting requirements and spend time on updates and reports about your project—if well-stewarded, many foundations and corporations will continue to support your work. If your grant request is rejected, inquire about why you were not funded and, if appropriate, request to resubmit your proposal after you have addressed the foundation's concerns. If the project has merit, consider approaching other foundations or individual donors with a similar plan tailored to their interests.

CONCLUSION—THE RESULTS OF PHILANTHROPY

The process of fundraising from individuals, corporations, and foundations allows you to create your advocacy vision for the future and to share that vision with others who have similar hopes and dreams. It requires you to think strategically about your program and define a manageable and measurable plan for the future. Because you know that donors are selflessly giving their resources to you, in return you feel compelled to be good stewards of their support. Since you are accountable to these donors, you spend their funding wisely, on the most critical needs of the program and on the areas that are in line with their interests. Through the process of inspiring donors, you are constantly reminded of the reasons you became involved in this work and you imagine your ideal future. Their confidence lifts you up when you feel less hopeful and their dedication fills you with promise. The end result of philanthropy at its best is a net gain for both you and the donor that far exceeds the dollar value of the gift itself.

REFLECTION QUESTIONS

1. As a health care professional, what sorts of ethical concerns do you have around fundraising from grateful patients? If a patient develops a closer relationship with a doctor as a result of their philanthropy and receives special treatment because of the relationship, does this cross ethical lines? How do you maintain patient confidentiality and abide by HIPPA regulations while fundraising?
2. What types of projects or activities do you feel would be more suitable for philanthropy from individuals? What activities do you feel would be more likely to be funded by corporations or foundations? Given the different funding motivations of each group, how would your messaging change if you were pitching a project to an individual, a corporation, or a foundation?
3. What are some of the ways you can identify good donor prospects from your health care practice? How can you let patients know about your work and invite them to get more involved? How can you articulate the needs of your program and the results of private funding?

PRACTICE MAKES PERFECT

1. An important part of philanthropy is articulating the needs of the organization and describing how you will use a donors funding with a measured impact. Imagine a donor has asked you for a

proposal for a $100,000, $1 million, or $10 million gift. Sketch out a brief budget and timeline for how you would use these funds. Write a two-paragraph justification that describes the funding need, the use, and what results you would expect to achieve.
2. When engaging a grateful patient in philanthropy, it is important to move at a respectful pace. You would not propose marriage on a first date and likewise you should not ask for a gift in the first meeting. Generally speaking, it takes five substantive interactions before a donor is willing to make a gift. Think about one of your grateful patients that might be interested in supporting your program and make a list of the ways you could educate them about your program and involve them further.
3. Create a list of potential foundations that are a match for your program and choose the top two that are most closely aligned. Spend some time researching each foundation on their website, look at their 90s, and search their mention in local publications. Draft a list of the ways that you match their interests and how you are uniquely positioned to achieve the best results. Use these points to craft a one-page letter of inquiry.
4. Sometimes when working with patients, they already understand the needs and benefits of your program. Other times you need to quickly be able to explain the complexities of the work you do in a meaningful and inspiring way. Using index cards, craft and rehearse your fundraising "elevator pitch" – how you would convince someone to support your program in during an elevator ride that lasts 60 seconds.

REFERENCES

Barret, V. (2010, July 23). Billionaire Marc Benioff: I'm sold: How the Salesforce. com CEO sold himself on giving away $100 million. *Forbes*. Retrieved July 30, 2011, from www.forbes.com/2010/07/22/salesforcecom-philanthropy-billionaires-intelligent-technology-marc-benioff.html

Charity 'Makes you feel better'. (2008, March 20). *BBC News*. Retrieved January 9, 2009, from http://news.bbc.co.uk/go/pr/fr/-/2/hi/health/7305395.stm

Callahan, D. (2008, January 31). A gentler capitalism: A sea of change may be afoot in how American business views its role in society. *Los Angeles Times*.

Campbell & Company Research Fellow. (2006). *Charitable giving to education, health and arts: An analysis of data collected in the center on philanthropy panel study, 2003*. Retrieved May 31, 2011, from www.campbellcompany.com/articles/

Caruso, D. (2008, January 6). Can foundations take the long view again? *The New York Times*. Business Section: RE: Framing.

Colorado Nonprofit Association. (2008). *Generous Colorado: Why donors give*. Retrieved May 31, 2011, from www.coloradononprofits.org/WhyDonorsGive/

Cornforth, S. (1999, May). Locking in corporate sponsorships. *Currents: Council for Advancement and Support of Education. XXV*(5), 46–47.
Dahnert, J. S. (1998, December). 12 ways to blow the ask. *Currents: Council for Advancement and Support of Education. XXIV.* Retrieved May 9, 2012, from www.case.org/Publications_and_Products/1998/NovemberDecember_1998/12_Ways_to_Blow_the_Ask.html
DiConsiglio, J. (2011, April). Arm in arm: Working closely with your board is essential to advancement. *Currents: Council for Advancement and Support of Education. XXXVII*(4), 14–20.
Duxbury, S. (2010, October 17). Benioffs' $100M UCSF gift raises hospital profile. *San Francisco Business Times.* Retrieved July 30, 2011, from www.bizjournals.com/sanfrancisco/stories/2010/10/18/focus7.html?surround=etf&ana=e_article&b=1287374400^4104421
Geever, J. C. *The foundation center's guide to proposal writing* (4th Edn). New York, NY: The Foundation Center, 2004.
Giving USA Foundation. (2010). *Giving USA 2010: The annual report on philanthropy for the year 2009.* Retrieved May 31, 2011, from www.givingusareports.org.
Guth, R. A. (2010, June 17). UCSF to Get $100 million for hospital: Gift from salesforce founder Benioff for children's center reflects rise of younger philanthropists from silicon valley. *The Wall Street Journal.* Retrieved July 30, 2011 from http://online.wsj.com/article/SB10001424052748704324304575307111971055670.html
Jarrell, A. (2005, May/June) Closing remarks: Novel ways. *Currents: Council for Advancement and Support of Education. XXXI*(5), 63–64.
King, R. (1989, June). Stating your case: The art, the science, and the future of the quintessential campaign document. *Currents: Council for Advancement and Support of Education. XV,* 46.
Kraus, R. J. (1998, February). The changing face of corporate giving. *Currents: Council for Advancement and Support of Education.*
Leonhardt, D. (2008, March 9). What makes people give? *The New York Times Magazine*: The Money Issue.
Mills, E. (2008, January). Doing philanthropy the Google way. *The New York Times.* Retrieved from www.CNET News.com
Rosso, H. A., & Tempel, E. R. (1991a). Chapter 2: Understanding the fund raising cycle. In *Achieving excellence in fundraising* (1st ed.). San Fransisco, CA: Jossey-Bass.
Rosso, H. A., & Tempel, E. R. (1991b). Chapter 17: How to research and analyze individual donors. In *Achieving excellence in fundraising* (1st ed.). San Fransisco, CA: Jossey-Bass.
Rosso, H. A., & Tempel, E. R. (1991c). Chapter 1: A philosophy of fundraising. In *Achieving excellence in fundraising* (1st ed.). San Fransisco, CA: Jossey-Bass.
The Foundation Center. (2011). *Demystifying the 990-PF.* Retrieved May 31, 2011, from http://foundationcenter.org/getstarted/tutorials/demystify/index.html
WealthEngine. (2010). *2010 healthcare report: Best practices for prospect research in healthcare fundraising.* Retrieved July 30, 2011, from www.scribd.com/doc/37873056/Best-Practices-for-Prospect-Research-in-Healthcare-Philanthropy-%E2%80%93–2nd-Edition

11

A Comprehensive Strategy: Putting It All Together

RICHARD L. BARNES

Never doubt that a small group of thoughtful, committed citizens can change the world. Indeed, it's the only thing that ever has.—Margaret Mead (American anthropologist, 1901–1978)

This final chapter is a case study of advocacy in action, an exhilarating example of successful public policy advocacy using the systematic approach to policy advocacy and the strategies and tactics described in this book. Thus far, you have learned how to weave educational principles with principled research. You understand how to cultivate relations with the media and use those for the benefit of liaising with legislators. You will see these approaches in this study, along with fundraising and the judicious use of law suits, which you now also understand. Above all, pay special attention to the collaboration among the coalition members and other key stakeholders that is key at every step of the way in this case study.

As you read this narrative, think to yourself about how daunting these achievements might have seemed just ten chapters ago. Try to identify ways in which you yourself might have helped to clear the smokescreen of corporate deception using the skills showcased here. How might you as an advocate fit into this web of working together for a common cause? Where do your own strengths lie? Talking with legislators? Writing up reports for news outlets? Raising money to keep up the fight?

THE PROBLEM

In 1987, legislation was making its way through the Oklahoma legislature that would have required nonsmoking areas in public places and workplaces, or allowed them to be entirely smoke-free, which was considered advanced for the time. The tobacco industry hijacked the bill, and the result was legislation that required smoking areas in all public places and workplaces, and prohibited cities from enacting stronger legislation (known as preemption). For the next 13 years, public health advocates in Oklahoma worked without success to undo the damage, but were unable to overcome the staunch opposition of the tobacco industry (Barnes & McCaffree, 2002). The tobacco industry cast its opposition as an economic battle, arguing, without any evidence to support it (and regularly rebutted by data), that forcing public venues, such as restaurants and bars, to be smoke-free would cause losses of 30% or more of their customers (Eriksen & Chaloupka, 2007; Scollo, Lal, Hyland, & Glantz, 2003).

The Tobacco-Free Oklahoma Coalition was formed in the mid-1990s, and consisted of the American Cancer Society, American Heart Association, American Lung Association, the State medical and dental associations and a few individuals, as well as the State health department as an ex officio member. The Coalition brought an organizational strength to the fray, but it was no more successful. So, how did the situation take a dramatic turn in 2000 with ultimate passage 3 years later of a very strong law that required most Oklahoma public places and workplaces to be smoke-free? Please read on!

FINDING PARTNERS: A COALITION IS REBORN

In November 1999, the Coalition elected two new leaders, a pulmonologist (Chair) and a lawyer/lobbyist (Vice Chair—Chair-Elect). The first order of business for the new leaders was to evaluate why there had been no progress in passing legislation to protect citizens from the known health hazards of secondhand tobacco smoke. The conclusion was that the Coalition: (a) did not have enough political clout to overcome the campaign contributions and lobbying prowess of the tobacco industry, (b) was not organized in a way that would maximize its effectiveness, (c) had a name connoting that its goal was to ban all tobacco, and (d) had not been aggressive enough.

In 2000, the Oklahoma legislature referred to voters a constitutional amendment to capture 75% of the millions of dollars a year in payments received by the state, as its share in the settlement of litigation by 46 states against the six major tobacco manufacturers under the 1998 Master Settlement Agreement (Givel & Glantz, 2004; National Association of Attorneys General) into a constitutional trust fund that would be free of legislative tinkering or defunding. The proposed amendment required that the money be spent on health, with particular emphasis on tobacco-related diseases. The successful campaign to pass the amendment generated a great deal of both paid and earned media attention on the impact of tobacco use on public health. The campaign organization for the amendment became the model for changing the Coalition.

The Coalition chair launched the OntracK Campaign (Oklahoma Tobacco Reduction and Cessation Campaign) in March 2000 to push for passage of SJR36, the legislation to refer the constitutional amendment to voters, and to press for smoke-free and other tobacco control legislation. The first step was to recruit a number of health care professional organizations as partners in the OntracK Campaign. By the end of the Legislative Session in May, the OntracK Campaign had played a major role in the passage of SJR36, and laws prohibiting smoking in all Oklahoma schools and creating the Tobacco Use Prevention and Cessation Revolving Fund to receive the 25% of the Master Settlement Agreement funds that would not go into the constitutional trust fund created by SJR36. The Revolving Fund was also to be expended on health programs.

The OntracK Campaign then played a significant role in securing the passage of the constitutional amendment by helping raise funds for the campaign and by conducting a media advocacy program using letters to the editor and editorial board meetings. After the successful election, the Coalition chair recruited all of the OntracK Campaign partners to join the Coalition.

The lasting legacy of the OntracK campaign was the refocusing of the tobacco control battle away from economics to public health. From that point forward, the Coalition was able to keep most of the media on the public health message in both reporting on the Coalition's legislative activities and in editorializing on the issues involved. And then came the surprise of 2000.

FORGING NEW, POWERFUL PARTNERSHIPS

While Coalition organizational changes were moving forward, an unexpected, new strategic opportunity was developing that the Coalition would later use to advance its legislative goals. In August 2000, the State Board of Health quietly requested a legal opinion from the Coalition Vice-Chair on the power of the Board to issue regulations prohibiting smoking in public places and workplaces. With an opinion in hand that the Board had such power, the Policy Committee of the Board began working on the regulations in late 2000, inviting the Coalition Vice-Chair to provide technical support for the process. While official Board activities are open to the public, Board members are appointed by the Governor and are not subject to the influence of lobbying and campaign contributions that the tobacco industry had successfully used to thwart the Coalition in the legislature. In June 2001, a new Commissioner of Health was selected by the Board of Health; he had come from the Florida Department of Health with experience in the very successful Florida tobacco control program. The new Commissioner was an outspoken foe of tobacco use, and became a lightning rod in the media battle. Neither the tobacco industry nor its allies participated in the proceedings of the Board of Health as it worked on the smoking regulations.

Meanwhile, the Coalition embarked on a process to systematically change the structure of the Coalition to foster an environment of full inclusion of all of the new partners recruited from the OntracK Campaign. Several surveys of partners' preferences were conducted that covered every aspect of Coalition activities including membership, leadership, and governance. In March 2001, a Restructuring Retreat was held to discuss and decide on implementation of change.

As the structural changes unfolded, a strategic plan was developed that covered all important issues in tobacco control in Oklahoma: smoke-free public places and workplaces, blocked youth access to tobacco products, smoking-cessation programs, and adequate funding for State and local tobacco control programs. In November 2001, the Coalition adopted a broad, detailed Strategic Plan for Clean Indoor Air in Oklahoma to work in parallel with the development of Board of Health regulations.

The Strategic Plan was based on polling data that showed substantial majority voter support for regulating smoking in public places and workplaces, including 31.1% support from smokers. The Plan called for an education program using the media to inform the public and business owners about the dangers of secondhand tobacco smoke, targeting of high-profile businesses permitting smoking by hand-billing customers and employees about the dangers of secondhand tobacco smoke, encouraging State and local governmental units to use existing laws to eliminate secondhand smoke exposures, assisting local governments in enacting ordinances restricting smoking to challenge the State preemption of local action, seeking repeal of statewide preemption, and, finally, passing a state law eliminating smoking in public places and workplaces. Over the next 18 months, every step of the Strategic Plan was executed, except for the targeting of high profile businesses.

In early 2002, the organization changed its name to the Oklahoma Alliance on Health or Tobacco to separate itself from the unsuccessful Coalition, and its membership climbed to about 30 organizations representing every health care professional organization in the state, along with several ethnic and regional tobacco control organizations and a well-positioned children's advocacy group. AARP joined the Alliance, which added a potent grassroots advocacy capability to the Alliance because of AARP's large membership. When it reached its peak membership in 2002, the combined membership of all of the organizations in the Alliance was equal to half of the voters in the 2000 gubernatorial election in Oklahoma, a fact the Alliance regularly mentioned to evidence its political clout, and a fact not lost on the political leadership at the Capitol.

An important tactical element of the new organization was a change in the way it used members' lobbyists and grassroots advocacy systems. Each organization with a lobbyist agreed to make the lobbyist available to the Alliance, and a protocol was developed to link the Alliance via e-mail to the grassroots coordinator of each of its members to facilitate the distribution of Action Alerts to members' grassroots advocates. The grassroots advocacy protocol would prove crucial in the passage of the 2003 legislation on smoking in public places and workplaces.

LEVERAGING PROGRESS: ON TO THE LEGISLATURE

The Alliance had sponsors introduce comprehensive smoke-free legislation in 2002 in companion bills in the Senate and the House, as it had in many previous years, prohibiting smoking in all public places and workplaces. Companion bills are identical in language and are often used to double the chances of success; if one passes, it has a better chance of passing in the opposite house. The Alliance also implemented its new lobbying strategy of having all its lobbyists meet at the capitol every Monday morning before the legislature went into session at 1:30 pm. Status reports were given and assignments were made to meet with specific legislators to gauge support for the bills and learn why there was or was not support.

For the first time since 1987 a measure of legislative success on smoke-free public places and workplaces was achieved; SB1553 was passed in April 2002 and signed into law to prohibit smoking in all state buildings. The road to victory was rocky and circuitous. SB1553 started as being comprehensive by prohibiting smoking in all public places and workplaces. By the time it crossed from the Senate to the House, it only prohibited smoking in the State capitol. When the bill was to be debated on the House floor, Alliance lobbyists, working with the House author, arranged for the bill to be called up for debate while its most vocal and influential member opposed to the bill was absent; he had a habit of coming back from lunch late. The House author offered a floor substitute that passed by a wide margin, and the Senate adopted the House amendments. This was a substantial victory as it covered thousands of State employees and all State venues including college dormitories, mental hospitals, and the prison system, a first for any state at the time. It set the stage for the argument in 2003 that State workers were not entitled to more protection than other workers.

The full Board of Health issued its final regulations in spring 2002. This was the turning point in the battle; the tobacco industry had no way to stop the issuance of the regulations, but it did attack the process in the media. The Alliance used the controversy to mount its own earned media effort in support of smoke-free public places and workplaces. Alliance leaders and the new Commissioner of Health briefed major newspapers' editorial boards, most of whom supported the Board's action. The news media provided extensive coverage of the issue.

As an integral part of its campaign to keep the news media framing the regulation of smoking as a public health issue, the Alliance had developed a manual of all of the peer-reviewed literature on the adverse health impacts of exposure to secondhand tobacco smoke, and on the real economics of smoke-free laws. Summaries of the journal articles were written that included the citations of the articles and the text of abstracts. The manuals were given to key reporters and all editorial boards. The summaries of the journal articles were given to all legislators. The manual became a key factor in getting and keeping extensive editorial board support for both the Board of Health regulations and the intense media campaign on the 2003 smoke-free public places and workplaces legislation.

The only way the tobacco industry could stop the implementation of the Board of Health regulations was to convince a majority in both houses of the legislature to disapprove them or to convince the Governor not to sign them. The Alliance had a substantial majority of support in the Senate, and had worked with the Governor's staff during the whole process to ensure that he would sign the regulations. A bill was filed in the House to disapprove the 2002 regulations, but was withdrawn before any action was taken on it.

For technical reasons, the Board of Health issued its 2002 regulations in two sets, one covering public places, including restaurants, and the other covering health care facilities. The Governor signed the second set, but declined to sign the set covering restaurants, finding a conflict with State law. However, the Governor urged the legislature to pass a law accomplishing what the regulations were designed to do. Taking that cue, the Alliance asked its legislative champions to find a bill that could be amended to do just that and SB696 became that vehicle. At this point, SB696 was in Conference Committee and had nothing to do with smoking, but when the Conference Committee Substitute emerged, it mirrored the Board of Health regulations that the Governor had rejected. The Conference Committee Substitute was rejected in the Senate and returned to Conference twice. The SB696 that finally passed both houses was identical to SB1553 that had passed a month earlier. The legislative fight was over for 2002, but the battle continued. Too late to fix the regulations problem before the 2002 Legislative Session ended at the end of May, the Board of Health issued emergency regulations in June that would expire when the 2003 Legislative Session began on the first Monday in February 2003.

FROM LEGISLATORS TO LAWSUITS

Once the emergency regulations went into effect in June 2002, the tobacco industry's front group, the Oklahoma Restaurant Association, filed a suit to block enforcement and obtained a restraining order to prevent enforcement. The tobacco industry has had a long history of using hospitality trade associations to "front" the tobacco industry's opposition to smoking restrictions, and built the alliance by convincing the hospitality industry that smoking restrictions would hurt their businesses (Dearlove, Bialous, & Glantz, 2002; Ritch & Begay, 2001). The lawsuit gave the Alliance an unexpected opportunity to keep the issue alive in the media until the legislature went into session in February 2003. To balance the fight, the American Lung Association filed a lawsuit in Federal court in July 2002 against the Restaurant Association on behalf of its constituents with lung conditions, who were seriously threatened by exposure to secondhand tobacco smoke and could not go into smoky environments; four of those constituents volunteered to be individual plaintiffs in the suit. The basis of the suit was a provision of the Americans with Disabilities Act that prohibits interference with the rights of the disabled, in this case persons with respiratory disabilities. In the end, the Restaurant Association suit became moot when the temporary rules expired in early February 2003, and the Lung Association dropped its suit because of that mootness. However, the value of the media attention that the lawsuits generated was incalculable.

To counter the Restaurant Association's economic claim that smoking restrictions would hurt business, through the summer 2002 into early 2003 the Alliance conducted a series of media events at restaurants that had gone smoke-free or had opened new smoke-free facilities to provide the media, the public, and legislators with testimonials from business owners and managers on why they made smoke-free decisions. During the media events, the Alliance representatives encouraged the media to interview customers about their views on smoking in restaurants; there was little risk in doing so as polling data showed a very high level of support for smoke-free restaurants. The media events were very well attended by electronic and print media outlets, and provided the Alliance with extensive coverage of the issue from July 2002 through the 2003 Legislative Session.

The Alliance had even brought about a reversal in the editorial position of the largest newspaper in the capital, after years of opposition, to strongly supporting tough restrictions on smoking. In large part, this was accomplished by working closely with the paper's health and capitol reporters, who were writing stories about the importance of the smoking restrictions to protect public health. It was a matter of convincing the editorial board that its position was in conflict with what the paper was reporting in the news.

A CONVERGENCE OF STRATEGIES, A FUMBLE, AND A SPRINT TO THE FINISH

As the Alliance prepared for the 2003 Legislative Session, it provided legislative sponsors with two bills that were filed in December 2002. Unlike prior years, the Alliance bills were different in several respects: HJR1011 called for a vote on a constitutional amendment to prohibit smoking in most public places and workplaces patterned after a successful voter-initiated, smoke-free constitutional amendment just passed in Florida in November 2002, and SB566 was legislation to achieve the same goal without a vote of the people.

The Oklahoma Restaurant Association had also secured the filing of a weaker Senate smoke-free bill, but its cosponsors were the two most powerful members of the legislature: the Senate President Pro-Tempore and the Speaker of the House. It also provided for submission of the issue to voters in a legislative referendum, an argument that the Association had been making in the media during the fall of 2002. When the 2003 Legislative Session opened on February 3, 2003, the Alliance had three very different measures to work with: a constitutional amendment, a legislative referendum, and straight legislation.

The decision was quickly made by the Alliance to focus on amending the Restaurant Association bill as it was likely to pass with such powerful sponsorship, and the Senate President Pro-Tempore was very supportive of the Alliance's goal. The Speaker of the House had never shown any interest in smoke-free legislation, either in support or opposition.

Passage of this bill, even with its powerful cosponsors and the work of the Restaurant Association and tobacco lobbyists to prevent the Board of Health from controlling the issue, was still not certain. The bill was weak and needed to be substantially changed, something the Restaurant Association did not want. The Alliance worked at solidifying the legislative support it had, and gaining new supporting legislators as the bill went through the committee process in the Senate. The Alliance also continued to press forward on its two measures because they were comprehensive, and there was no assurance that the Restaurant Association bill could be fixed.

11 A Comprehensive Strategy: Putting It All Together

The Alliance adopted a slogan for the legislative campaign, "It's About Health, and It's About Time," and passed out political-style buttons; some legislators wore them. A logo with the slogan appeared on press releases and material delivered to legislators' offices.

Passing legislation is a process of fits and starts. There is a flurry of activity when a legislative committee is holding hearings on a bill or a house is conducting debate on a bill, and then quiet. The Alliance lobbyists met every Monday morning whether any action on any of the bills was scheduled for that week or not. There was much work to do to canvas legislators to sound out their support for the bills. Legislators' questions about the need for the legislation required answers. Getting a bill passed is a full-time endeavor, and the Alliance's lobbyists worked at it full time. Regular visits were made to the print and electronic media offices in the capitol; reporters were always looking for something new to report on this contentious issue.

On March 31, 2003, the Board of Health reissued its 2002 emergency regulations covering restaurants and other public places. Here the Alliance dropped the ball. A new Governor had taken office in January 2003, and there was no serious lobbying of the Governor's Office like that carried out with the previous Governor. As a result, the new Governor rejected the regulations on May 15, 2003, but called on the legislature to enact tough restrictions on smoking in public places. At this point, all three of the original measures were very much alive and were in Conference Committees, but the focus of the Alliance was on the Restaurant Association bill.

The Alliance was successful in taking control of the process. The Restaurant Association bill was amended several times in the Senate, and it didn't look like it could pass in the House. The goal of the Alliance was to get the bill out of the House intact and go to a Conference Committee of members of both houses who would negotiate a final version of the bill. The Alliance engineered a technical procedural amendment in the House to pass it without a vote on the merits of the legislation. The Senate rejected the House amendment sending it to Conference Committee, where members of both houses hammered out the final language. It was at this point that the support of the Senate President Pro-Tempore became crucial—he demanded that the Restaurant Association lobbyist work out the final language with the Alliance in a marathon meeting in his office.

In the marathon meeting, the Restaurant Association lobbyist let it slip that the Association's only issue was delaying the implementation of the law in restaurants for as long as possible. The Restaurant Association proposed 5 years, the Alliance countered with 18 months, and 30 months was finally agreed to. Everything fell into place and the Alliance got everything else it wanted in the Conference Committee Substitute.

However, there was now only 1 week left before mandatory adjournment of the Legislative Session, and the bill had to pass again in both houses. It easily passed the Senate 3 days before adjournment, 36-9, but it was still not clear how it would do in the House as the merits had not been tested. The Alliance had heavily lobbied House members since the session had begun; the media campaign had been intense with significant editorial support for the bill.

With 2 days left, the bill was called up in the House in the morning, but failed 47:51. A notice to reconsider the bill later that day was filed, and the value of the Alliance' grassroots advocacy system was proven. E-mail action alerts were sent out immediately after the morning vote; only three Nays had to be changed to Ayes to carry the day. The Alliance asked for help from the Republican Lieutenant Governor to work members of her party, who had largely voted Nay, and the bill was passed 3 hours later, 52:45.

A RECAP: LESSONS LEARNED

In the case study above, success was achieved because of the combination of strategic and tactical moves by the Alliance. The first was the complete restructuring of the advocacy partnership into the Alliance. Next, it was taking the fight out of the legislature, where the tobacco industry had heavy clout, to the State Board of Health, where it had no clout. Success there put the tobacco industry and its ally, the Restaurant Association, on the defensive. The lawsuit by the Restaurant Association gave the Alliance the opportunity to keep the issue in the news between Legislative Sessions, usually a dead zone on legislative issues. Once the Board of Health regulations were issued, the Alliance knew that the Restaurant Association was desperate for legislation that it could play a role in crafting to negate the Board of Health regulations. That desperation gave the Alliance significant leverage in negotiations for the final bill, aided by its supporter: the Senate President Pro-Tempore. In an unscientific poll after the bill was passed, Alliance lobbyists queried legislators' staff on phone calls, e-mails, and faxes in support of the bill that last day; nearly every one reported being contacted in one or more forms in support of the bill. In the final fight for the bill in the House, it was the coordinated lobbying and grassroots advocacy system that the Alliance had crafted that carried the day.

In late 2003, a new coalition was formed to work on legislation to fight childhood obesity. It replicated the Alliance in every way, and all of the members of the Alliance on Health or Tobacco joined the new Oklahoma Fit Kids Alliance. In 2005, the Fit Kids Alliance achieved its initial legislative goals on school nutrition despite strong opposition from the high fructose corn syrup beverage and the vending machine industries.

EPILOGUE

All that's necessary for the forces of evil to win in the world is for enough good men to do nothing. — Edmund Burke (British orator, philosopher, and politician, 1729–1797)

Now that you can see that the process of advocacy is not really so mysterious, complex, or daunting, what are you waiting for? In answering that question, keep this in mind: In providing patient care, you are impacting one life at a time; by changing health policy through political advocacy, you can impact thousands of lives.

With what you have learned from reading this book, you are now prepared for a lifelong habit of civic engagement. You will find it unexpectedly rewarding.

REFERENCES

Barnes, R., & McCaffree, D. R. (2002). Tobacco wars—The physician's role in public health advocacy. *Journal of the Oklahoma State Medical Association, 95*(3), 120–125.

Dearlove, J. V., Bialous, S. A., & Glantz, S. A. (2002). Tobacco industry manipulation of the hospitality industry to maintain smoking in public places. *Tobacco Control, 11*(2), 94–104.

Eriksen, M., & Chaloupka, F. (2007). The economic impact of clean indoor air laws. *CA Cancer Journal for Clinicians, 57*(6), 367–378.

Givel, M. & Glantz, S. A. (2004). The "global settlement" with the tobacco industry: 6 years later. *American Journal of Public Health, 94*(2), 218–224.

National Association of Attorneys General (1998). *Master Settlement Agreement.* Retrieved July, 2011, from www.naag.org/backpages/naag/tobacco/msa/msa-pdf

Ritch, W. A., & Begay, M. E. (2001). Strange bedfellows: The history of collaboration between the Massachusetts Restaurant Association and the tobacco industry. *American Journal of Public Health, 91*(4), 598–603.

Scollo, M., Lal, A., Hyland, A., & Glantz, S. (2003). Review of the quality of studies on the economic effects of smoke-free policies on the hospitality industry. *Tobacco Control, 12*(1), 13–20.

Appendix

Introduction

Congratulations! You have worked your way through this textbook and, we hope, have envisioned many ways to use practical techniques for successful advocacy on behalf of individual patients and patient populations. You have also seen numerous case examples throughout the book that exemplify how others have used the tactics and strategies described in every chapter.

This appendix contains a few more examples of successful advocacy. We have carefully selected these examples in order to further demonstrate both specific skills that individual advocates have used and the blending of many approaches by multiple stakeholders collaborating on behalf of a common purpose. As you learn from these examples, activate your own learning by asking yourself which skills from this textbook are at work, and try to imagine yourself employing them as these advocates have done. Your chance to channel them toward your our advocacy goals begins now!

Media Case Study

A Trio of Twitter Tales

PIERRETTE MIMI POINSETT

A PHYSICIAN'S RESPONSE TO A SIGNIFICANT PRICE CHANGE IN A PHARMACEUTICAL

In March, the FDA awarded KV Pharmaceutical orphan drug approval to package 17 hydroxyprogesterone (170P) as Makena. This product had been used for many years in a compounded form by obstetricians to prevent preterm delivery. With the introduction of Makena, the price of a single dose increased from $10 (in the generic compound) to $1,500 ($30,000 per price tag). Additionally KV Pharmaceutical sent out warning letters to compounding pharmacies to cease production of the compounded generic version.

Obstetrician Dr. Jen Gunter, and author of the *The Preemie Primer* (Gunter, 2010), began blogging and tweeting about this price increase and its impact on cost and access to care. As a result, Makena became a trending topic on Twitter. Other physicians, nurses, health advocates, and parent tweeters picked up the topic to continue the dialogue. Three congresspersons also began investigations and made contact with the pharmaceutical company. Consumers created Facebook pages about the Makena issue that "went viral." Dr. Gunter reports that she was interviewed multiple times by national and local press. With increasing public pressure, KV Pharmaceutical dropped the price of their product. Compounding pharmacies were also able to continue producing generic versions of 170P.

A GRASSROOTS NONPROFIT WITH A STRONG SOCIAL MEDIA BASE

MomsRising is a grassroots movement that describes itself as a "nonprofit organization working to build family-friendly America." Since 2006, this organization has actively utilized social media, leveraging targeted newsletters, electronic petitioning, and tweeting. Key to their success has been frequent tweet chats about issues including paid sick leave, health care access, and toxic phthalates. During 2010, MomsRising members took over a million actions in support of families and were covered extensively by the media. Changing Internal Revenue Service (IRS) policy on breast pumps and breastfeeding supplies was a major campaign success for MomsRising. In the fall of 2010, the IRS determined that "breastfeeding does not have enough health benefits to qualify as a form of medical care" and as a result would not allow breast pumps and supplies to be purchased using funds in pre-tax medical accounts. MomsRising initiated an electronic petition campaign in addition to frequent blog posting, tweeting, and tweet chats about the IRS policy.

A lively response ensued, bringing together concerned family members, other child advocacy organizations, and professional societies involved in the care and welfare of children. These discussions spread throughout the internet, including *The New York Times* website, Facebook, Twitter, and other discussion boards. The IRS received letters signed by 41 House and Senate members detailing the health and medical benefits of breastfeeding. Meanwhile, 24,000 MomsRising participants signed an electronic petition calling on the IRS to reverse their decision. The IRS reversed its decision in February 2011, making breast pumps and supplies eligible for medical savings account funds (MomsRising, 2011).

ZOMBIE APOCALYPSE: ENGAGING YOUNG ADULTS ABOUT DISASTER PREPAREDNESS

In May of 2011, the Centers for Disease Control and Prevention (CDCP) launched a media campaign to prepare for the start of hurricane season. The campaign also benefitted from an evangelical minister's prediction of the end of the world on May 21, 2011. The blog post started off by referencing "Zombie Apocalypse," a popular video game and movie theme. Normally CDCP blogs receive 2,000–3,000 hits in total. Prior to this social campaign the most popular CDCP blog received 10,000 hits (Reuters, 2011). Within 2 days, the "Zombie Apocalypse" blog had 60,000 hits, crashing the blog server. The topic went viral and became a trending topic on Twitter. For the first time the CDCP was able to successfully engage a media savvy demographic.

These three Twitter examples highlight the versatility of Twitter. Advocates can use Twitter to broadcast original content as well as to curate content. They can engage partners and stakeholders informally to amplify a message. They can facilitate dialogue via Tweet chats in real time, using hashtags* to follow a conversation. Twitter feeds can also be linked to a webinar, podcast, blog talk, radio, or live face-to-face conferences to enhance audience participation.

REFERENCES

Gunter, J. (2010). *The preemie primer: A complete guide for parents of premature babies—from birth through the toddler years and beyond.* Cambridge, MA: Da Capo Lifelong Books.

MomsRising. (2011). *Victory for moms, babies & breastpumps: Good job, IRS!* Retrieved October 12, 2011, from www.momsrising.org/blog/victory-for-moms-babies-breastpumps-good-job-irs/

Reuters. (2011). *CDC launches "Zombie Apocalypse" disaster preparedness campaign.* Retrieved October 12, 2011, from www.ktla.com/news/landingktla-cdc-zombie-apocalypse-preparedness,0,6033341.story

---

*As defined by Twitter (https://support.twitter.com/articles/49309-what-are-hashtags-symbols), the "#" symbol, called a "hashtag," is used to mark keywords or topics in a Tweet. It was created organically by Twitter users as a way to categorize messages. People use the hashtag symbol before relevant keywords in their Tweets so that they show more easily in Twitter Search. Clicking on a hashtagged word in any message shows you all other Tweets in that category. Hashtags can occur anywhere in the Tweet. Hashtagged words that become very popular are often "Trending Topics."

Research Case Study

Edgewood's Kinship Support Network: Using Research Findings to Develop a Community Program

DONALD COHON

THE PROBLEM

Foster child placement with relatives, known as kinship care, grew dramatically in the late 1980s and early 1990s creating a particular burden among grandparents in the African American community (Dubowitz, Feigelman, & Zuravin, 1993; Minkler, Roe, & Price, 1992; Thornton, 1991). States' policies for kinship care have been reviewed as reactive, "influenced more by the increasing demand for placement services and the decreasing number of available foster homes than by a societal commitment to the importance of relatives in the lives of abused, neglected and dependent children" (Gleeson & Craig, 1994, p. 26). Needless to say, the well-being of burdened grandparents was also a significant problem. This case study demonstrates the use of research to advocate on behalf of this group and use data to improve services.

Edgewood Center for Children and Families (Edgewood) is the leading provider of mental health and social services for children and families in crisis in San Francisco and San Mateo counties. Our mission is to strengthen children, youth, families, and their communities through service, training, advocacy, and research. Edgewood was founded in 1851 to provide a safe haven for orphans during the Gold Rush. Grandparents Who Care (GWC) was founded in 1989 to support grandparents stressed by the responsibility of caring for their grandchildren. In early 1992, Edgewood's Director of Program Development (DPD) was invited to attend a GWC support group of predominantly (90%) African American kinship caregivers with the aim of conducting a needs assessment and shifting the program's management to Edgewood.

Typically, aging African Americans rely on their children and grandchildren who have attained comparatively greater levels of education and have more interaction with mainstream society (Luckey, 1994). But support from these immediate kin for GWC grandparents was often not available because of problems experienced by the second and/or third generations (e.g., substance abuse, mental illness, AIDS). As familial networks of support erode, these now caregiving grandparents become more isolated and dependent on public bureaucracies for support, rather than more typical, informal family supports. But Edgewood's needs assessments had shown that unfamiliarity with and mistrust of the formal public service system inhibits kin caregivers from seeking the assistance they need from these public agencies.

Over the course of a year, the DPD transcribed caregivers' concerns and refined these qualitative data into three predominant themes expressing needs for respite from caregiving responsibilities, recreational activities for children, and respect for the caregivers from agency caseworkers. In March 1993, the Director of Edgewood's Institute for the Study of Community-Based Services conducted a formal needs assessment of GWC kinship caregivers using an instrument based on the Family Needs Scale (FNS) (Dunst, Trivette, & Deal, 1988). This research tool elicited an expanded set of needs:

- Respite
- Money
- Peer support
- Increased with their grandchildren's behavioral problems, including drug use
- Increased understanding of public agencies' bureaucracies, including the practice of having two or three caseworkers involved from the same agency
- Getting to know their caseworkers, who just "run in and out"

To begin a new program required start-up support, and initial advocacy efforts using these data were focused internally to Edgewood, that is, convincing the Board of Directors to use their own private agency funds to initiate the program. Kin caregivers lobbied individual Board members and brought them to the GWC support groups. When the issue was presented at the Board of Directors meeting, several kin caregivers were present to further substantiate the qualitative and quantitative data analyses. The Board voted to support the start up of the program.

Next, Edgewood used these data in discussions with the San Francisco Department of Social Services (now Human Services Agency, SFHSA) and San Francisco Community Mental Health Services (SFCMHS) to successfully advocate for the creation of the Kinship Support Network (KSN). Having these data from the outset of the program provided important insights into improving services and gave KSN a valuable educational tool to use with policy makers.

From the outset, kin caregivers themselves were part of the advocacy strategy, attending community meetings and also meetings of the commissioners of the SFHSA with whom Edgewood was negotiating a contract to provide support to these grandparents.

The KSN model is an example of a contractual, community-based service approach with the public Department of Homeland Security (DHS) acting as a "managed care" agency by monitoring services. KSN's primary mission is to provide a comprehensive, private-sector response and to offer case-managed services that fill gaps in public social services. This privatized model delivers services at the community level without evident participation in a public sector program, which caregivers had indicated they found stigmatizing. At the same time, the KSN model also gives the public agencies (in this case, SFHSA and SFCMHS) sufficient oversight and controls to ensure that mandated policies are observed. High caseloads at public agencies and lack of culturally informed staff inhibit outreach efforts to the kin caregiver community. To bridge this gap and also address the mistrust of public agencies elicited in the data gathering phase, KSN hired elderly African American and Latino grandparents from the communities where kinship caregivers live. With training and supervision these paraprofessional Community Workers (CW) effectively link, monitor, and provide advice to caregiver clients, assuming the roles of the second and third generations in the informal extended family support system.

Using data collected since the program's inception, KSN approached legislators about the circumstances of these kin caregivers and was able to present positive preliminary findings that were subsequently published showing reduction of needs on the modified FNS (Cohon & Cooper, 1999). These legislative meetings resulted in the passage of AB1193 (Kinship Support Services Act, 1997) that named Edgewood as the model for kinship care in California law for other California counties implementing similar programs. Even today, Edgewood has a contract with the California Department of Social Services (CDSS) to provide technical assistance to over 30 Kinship Supportive Services Projects (KSSP) in 20 California counties. In 2000, Edgewood expanded its KSN model to the agency's San Mateo office. Kin caregivers continue to be involved in advocating with county agencies and coupled with ongoing dissemination of data both directly to county agencies and in professional journals, KSN has had multi-year contracts with both San Francisco and San Mateo counties for provision of kinship services.

THE RESULTS

Since its inception, San Francisco KSN has provided services to 1,428 kin caregivers, 1,324 (92.7%) of whom are women, with an average age of 66. The program has served 2,985 children with an average current age of 8.3

and a standard deviation of 5.2 years. Of this number 1,461 (48.9%) were female. The majority totaling 1,693 (56.7%) are grandchildren. Since 2000, in neighboring San Mateo County, KSN has provided services to 1,017 kin caregivers with an average age of 57, 916 (90.1%) of whom are women. The program has served 2,808 children with an average current age of 8.6 and a standard deviation of 5.3 years. Of this number 1,322 (47.1%) were female. Again, grandchildren comprise the largest category: 1,091 (38.9%). Racial distributions for kin caregivers and foster children are shown in the table below.

County	African American	Asian	Latino/ Hispanic	Caucasian	Other
San Francisco kin caregivers	672 (47.1%)	135 (9.5%)	114 (8.0%)	47 (3.3%)	460 (32.2%)
San Francisco children	1,626 (54.5%)	151 (5.1%)	264 (8.8%)	55 (1.8%)	889 (29.7%)
San Mateo kin caregivers	326 (32.1%)	20 (2.0%)	282 (27.7%)	235 (23.1%)	154 (15.1%)
San Mateo children	798 (28.4%)	375 (13.4%)	938 (33.4%)	445 (15.8%)	252 (8.9%)

Since KSN began providing services, the Institute Director successfully sought public and private grant support for the program. Because of the data that continue to be collected by both sites, Edgewood's KSN has received funding support from the National Center on Child Abuse and Neglect, the Children's Bureau Administration on Children and Families, the Department of Justice's Office of Juvenile Justice, Delinquency Prevention, California's Office of Criminal Justice Planning, the Robert Wood Johnson Foundation, the California Endowment, the David and Lucile Packard Foundation, the California Wellness Foundation, the Zellerbach Family Fund, the William Randolph Hearst Foundation, and the Stuart Foundations. The most recent grant received was in 2009 from the Department of Health and Human Services' (HHS) Administration for Children and Families for $1.5 million over a period of 3 years to develop and implement the Kinship Support Network Navigator Program (KSNNP).

REFERENCES

Cohon, D., & Cooper, A. B. (1999). Edgewood's kinship support network: Program model and client characteristics. *Children and Youth Services Review, 21*(4), 311–338.

Dubowitz, H., Feigelman, S., & Zuravin, S. (1993). A profile of kinship care. *Child Welfare, 72*, 153–169.

Dunst, C. J., Trivette, C. M., & Deal, A. G. (1988). *Enabling and empowering families: Principles and guidelines for practice.* Cambridge, MA: Brookline Books.

Gleeson, J. P., & Craig, L.C. (1994). Kinship care in child welfare: An analysis of states' policies. *Children and Youth Services Review, 16*(1/2), 7–31.

Luckey, I. (1994, February). African American elders: The support network of generational kin. *Families in Society: The Journal of Contemporary Human Services,* 82–89.

Minkler, M., Roe, K. M., & Price, M. (1992). The physical and emotional health of grandmothers raising grandchildren in the crack cocaine epidemic. *Gerontologist, 32,* 752–761.

Thornton, J. L. (1991). Permanency planning for children in kinship foster homes. *Child Welfare, LXX*(5), 593–601.

Community Organizations Case Study

Partners in Health's Mental Health Program in Haiti: How an Initial Crisis Led to Advocacy for a Critical Unmet Need, an Expanded Program, Organizational Change, and a Shared National Mental Health Planning Effort

GIUSEPPE RAVIOLA, CATHERINE OSWALD,
AND FATHER EDDY EUSTACHE

THE PROBLEM

Significant challenges exist in developing a systematic approach to advocacy in the setting of an unforeseen disaster. While the role of the advocate can be one of overcoming opposition to change, doing so in an international context, in a situation of dramatic human loss, precipitous social change, and multiple competing needs, can present particularly difficult decisions and ethical dilemmas. This case describes the experience of transnational team members of an international health care organization who used an initial emergency response after the 2010 Haiti earthquake to advocate for immediate mental health care along with greater organizational commitment and a national planning effort for long-term mental health services.

THE CONTEXT

Zanmi Lasante (ZL), founded in 1983, provides health care in Haiti's Central Plateau and Artibonite Valley with a staff of approximately 5,000 providers, including 2,500 Community Health Workers (CHWs) through 11 hospitals in partnership with the Haitian Ministry of Health (also known as Ministère de la Santé Publique et de la Population, or MSPP). For more than 25 years, ZL has collaborated with Partners in Health (PIH), an international health care organization founded in Haiti in 1987 and based in Boston that works in 12 countries. PIH works to strengthen collaboration between nongovernmental organizations (NGOs) and local public systems in order to facilitate sustainable approaches and local capacity building. In January 2010, a major earthquake struck Haiti crumbling the city of Port-au-Prince and causing massive casualties. PIH's experience in health care delivery and program implementation in Haiti enabled it to be among the first responders to the medical crises following the earthquake. Prior to the earthquake the ZL psychosocial programs were developed to focus primarily on socioeconomic, educational, and psychological needs of children and families affected by HIV/AIDS and tuberculosis; these served as a platform upon which to expand dedicated mental health services following the disaster. With regard to mental health, PIH had only a nascent program.

ADVOCACY EFFORTS

In the weeks following the earthquake a small group comprised of Haitian and U.S. nationals within the organization began to advocate both within and outside the organization for mounting a sustained mental health service response to the disaster. Immediate linkages were made with like-minded organizations in Haiti that had some experience. In the first month following the earthquake initial needs assessments were completed, including surveys of current services within and outside of ZL and through meetings with Haitian mental health service leaders. A month after the earthquake, representatives of that team met with the Minister of Health for Haiti, facilitated by PIH's medical director. At that meeting the Minister acknowledged that the mental health needs of the population had been neglected prior to the earthquake, and requested the organization's support in developing a national mental health response to the disaster. The team proposed an effort by which the organization would use an initial organizational response as a foundation for a sustained, longer-term organizational commitment to development of mental health services, and for the development of a model community-based mental health care structure that would be shared with the Ministry, as part of a broader planning effort organized and led by the Ministry.

The team advocated internally for a significantly increased commitment to mental health services. This included initial lobbying of the organization's leadership, and external advocacy to foundations for start-up support of services. PIH added a new Boston-based mental health director, an adult and child psychiatrist, to support the Haitian team. In the 6 months following the earthquake, PIH/ZL expanded capacity to deliver mental health and psychosocial services through its programs by hiring additional staff and bringing staffing numbers to 17 psychologists (from three) and 50 social workers and social work assistants (from 20).

The team understood that building mental health systems of care in Haiti in the context of the disaster would require a systematic, integrated, evidence-based, and multi-sectoral approach, as well as cooperation and expertise beyond what any one organization, institution, or government could provide. In the weeks after the earthquake PIH/ZL began meeting biweekly in Port-au-Prince with representatives from other organizations in the United Nations cluster group process to plan and strategize. In collaboration with MSPP, the World Health Organization, and the Pan-American Health Organization (PAHO), PIH/ZL worked with other organizations to encourage a process that would lead to the drafting of a national plan for decentralized mental health services. Early in the process PIH/ZL offered the group some suggestions for the care pathways upon which a national mental health plan could potentially be developed.

Following PIH/ZL's increased service commitment, they teamed up with patients who benefited from mental health care. Alongside clinicians, patients advocated for the importance of these services by speaking openly about their positive treatment experiences in the community and to the medical system. Patients with preexisting mental illness prior to the earthquake who received care spoke about how it helped them to reintegrate into meaningful community activities such as church, choir, and school. The improvement of their social functioning reduced stigma and informed not only members of the community but also organizational medical staff, most of whom had never received formal mental health training. Efforts by the PIH communications team to share the stories of these patients in a nonstigmatizing way raised awareness within and beyond the organization's administrative structure about the initial successes of mental health care delivered by PIH/ZL.

By 6 months after the earthquake a proposal was developed for a systematic, collaborative process leading to the development of a scalable model for development of safe, effective, community-based, and culturally sound mental health services in the ZL system. This proposal was presented to potential funders, with a clear programmatic financial commitment having already been made by PIH/ZL to mental health service delivery. PIH leaders were recruited to advocate for foundational support toward this endeavor. Despite the limited human resource capacity of the mental health team, within a year after the earthquake several academic publications and research proposals had been developed and submitted.

THE RESULTS

At one and one-half years after the earthquake, ZL staff had provided approximately 20,000 individual services for mental health needs. Buy-in of organizational leadership permitted the formal integration of mental health into the health system strengthening the mission of the organization, now with the ZL and PIH Mental Health programs having their own structures and dedicated budgets.

Initial public and private grant support was obtained through active engagement with the PIH development and communications teams, and organizations expressing interest in post-earthquake mental health services. The Digicel Foundation and One x One provided support for the systems-building proposal, which integrated the collective strengths of a Haiti-based NGO (ZL), a social science research group (the Interuniversity Institute for Research and Development, INURED), MSPP, and several U.S.-based academic medical centers. As a result, a qualitative study of local beliefs and perceived needs in the community was completed, leading to the creation of a screening tool for mental disorders for use by CHWs. Through dedicated foundational support and internal financial commitments, a stepped care model for mental health services with articulation of provider tasks along a continuum of care is being developed, with accompanying treatment algorithms, decision supports, training and curriculum products, outcomes measurement tools, and provision of long-term planning support to MSPP. NIMH has funded an R21 feasibility study to develop research capacity through ZL, focused on a school-based mental health intervention in Haiti's Central Plateau.

In June 2011, a conglomerate of organizations met under the leadership of MSPP and WHO/PAHO to convene planning on a shared strategy for a national mental health plan. PIH/ZL employed a full-time psychiatrist in Haiti to support the training needs of an expert Haitian clinical team in mental health services to be based at the new PIH flagship hospital at Mirebalais, which in the future will receive most Haitian university medical trainees. In October 2011, MSPP and ZL/PIH observed World Mental Health Day for the second consecutive year under the banner "With a clear mind, your body is stronger (Ak tèt klè kò a pi djanm)."

Index

Accreditation Council for Graduate Medical Education (ACGME), 15
Activism, 2, 3
Administrative Procedure Act, 114
Administrative rulemaking, 29, 30, 37, 40
Advanced care, planning for, 92–93, 97
Advisory council, 172–173
"Advocacy Day," 149
Advocacy imperative, 13–14
Aged population, evidenced-based practices in, 123–124
Alberghetti v. Corbis Corp., 112
Albert Schweitzer Fellowship, 8–9
Amchem Products, Inc. v. Windsor, 1997, 110
American Academy of Child and Adolescent Psychiatry (AACAP), 149
American Dental Association (ADA), 2
American Lung Association, 182, 187
American Medical Association (AMA), 2
American Nurse's Association (ANA), 2
American Psychiatric Association (APA), 78–79
American's With Disabilities Act (ADA), 114
Association of American Medical Colleges (AAMC), 3
Attorney–client relationship, 111–112
Audience response system, 23
Audiences, understanding, 69

Ausiello, Dennis, 3
Autism Advocate, 151
Autism Society of America (ASA) (case study), 145–146, 150–151

Becker and Geer's study, 4–5
Bill, passing, 54, 188
Bill becoming law, 37, 52–56
Bill of rights for children with mental health disorders and their families (case study), 148–149
Blogs, 77
Brenner, Jeff, 125–126

California Subclass, 116
Causes of action, examples of, 114–115
Cerebral palsy, child with (case study), 88–89
Claims, 106–107
Class action, 105
  class certification, 107
  examples of causes, 114–115
  Federal Rule of Civil Procedure, 107–114
  history and policies behind class actions, 106
  Klay V. Humana, Inc. (case study), 115–119
  reasons for, 106–107
  types of, 114
  versus individual action, 106
  working, 107

Index

Class certification, 107, 113
  Federal Rules of Civil Procedure, 107–114
Class representatives, 107, 108–110, 111, 112
  duties of, 109
Clayton Act, 115
Collaborations, 144–145
  avoiding problems in, 150
  with community organizations, 149–150
  successful, 143, 145
"Colleagues in Caring," 134, 137
Commonality, 108, 110
Common questions, predominance of, 110
Commonwealth Fund Report (2007), 13
Community organizations, 146–147. *See also* Families and community organizations
  case study, 202–205
  collaborating with, 149–150
  identifying and approaching, 147–148
Companion legislation, 54
Consol. Rail Corp. v. Town of Hyde Park, 1995, 107–108
Constituent, 43–44, 59, 77
Continuing medical education (CME), 18
Corporations and funding, 159
Corporations fundraising, 175–177
  inquiry/proposal to, 176–177
Cultivation and involvement, in fundraising, 165–166
Cynicism, 4, 5

Digital realm, 76
Disability benefit denials, 90
Donor relationships, maintaining, 170–171

Earned media versus paid media, 68–69
Editorial boards, 42–43, 70, 186, 188
Editors
  contacts with, 71
  letters to, 73–74
Education

Accreditation Council for Graduate Medical Education (ACGME), 15
continuing medical education (CME), 18
graduate medical education (GME), 15
Internet-based continuing medical education (CME), 19
strategies that do not work, 17–18
strategies that work, 19–21
undergraduate medical education (UME), 15
as unmet legal needs, 87–89, 95
Elaborate new knowledge, 20
Elected officials, 40, 44, 57, 58
Electronic Communications Privacy Act, 115
E-mail, 70
Emotional information, 43
Employment
  as unmet legal needs, 89–90, 96
ERISA Class, 116
"Ethical erosion," 4
Eviction defense (case study), 86
Evidence-based policy design, 34
  designing the new policy, 36–39
  using scientific research in advocacy, 34–36
Executive branch head, 44
Executive Committee, 33
Expert speakers, 58

Facebook, 77
Face time, 58
Factual information, 43
Families and community organizations, 143
  advocacy odyssey and message for health professionals (case study), 153–155
  Autism Society of America (ASA) (case study), 145–146, 150–151
  bill of rights for children with mental health disorders and their families (case study), 148–149
  collaboration, 149–150
  health professional, participation of, 146–147
  identifying and approaching, 147–148

Index

MIND Institute, development of (case study), 152–153
  parent/family organizations as partners, 144–145
Family/parent groups, collaborating with, 144–145
Farmer, Paul, 3
"The Fate of Idealism in Medical School," 4–5
Federal Information Security Management Act of 2002 (FISMA), 115
Federal legislation, 38
Federal legislative process, 56
Federal Rules of Civil Procedure, 107–114
  after certification, 113
  appointment of lead counsel, 111
  commonality, 108
  notice and opting out, 112–113
  numerosity, 107–108
  predominance of common questions, 110
  resolution of the case, 113–114
  role of class counsel, 111–112
  superiority of case management, 110–111
  typicality, 108–110
Federal Senators, 53
Federal Statutes, 114–115
Feedback, 20
Filibuster, 54
First reading, 54
Food and utilities (case study), 84
Formal rule change, 101
The Foundation Center, 175
Foundation fundraising, 175–177
  inquiry/proposal to, 176–177
Foundations and funding, 158–159
F.T.C. v. Anheuser-Busch, Inc., 1960, 115
Funding, for researches, 125–127
Funds, finding, 157
  foundations and corporations, 175–177
  fundraising from individuals, 161–163
    cultivation and involvement, 165–166
    development lifecycle, 163
    identification and qualification, 163–164
    solicitation, 168–169
    strategy, planning, 164–165
  fundraising roles and responsibilities, 159–161
  private donors, 173–175
  sources, 157–159
  volunteers, 172–173

Genetic Information Nondiscrimination Act of 2008, 115
Global Class, 116
GovTrack, 60
Graduate medical education (GME), 15
Grassroots advocacy, 34
GuideStar, 175

Hanlon v. Chrysler Corp. (1998), 109
Hansberry v. Lee, 1940, 109
Health care in the United States, 1
Health care professionals
  in donors identification, 163–164
Health care reform, implementation of, 125
Health care system, 13
Health Insurance Portability and Accountability Act (HIPPA), 115
Health professionals
  and community organization, 146–147
Health professions
  promoting advocacy from within and from outside, 6–9
HJR1011, 188
"Hopper," 53
Hospital readmissions, prevention of, 126
House of God, 5
Housing
  as unmet legal needs, 85–87, 95

Idealism
  and advocacy, 3–6
  definition of, 3
IHELP, 82
Importance of advocacy, 1–2
Income, as unmet legal needs, 83–84, 94
Individual action, versus class action, 106

210 Index

Individuals, fundraising from, 158–159, 161–163
  cultivation and involvement, 165–166
  identification and qualification, 163–164
  solicitation, 168–169
  strategy, planning, 164–165
Inner advocate, discovering, 1
  idealism and advocacy, 3–6
  importance of advocacy, 1–2
  promoting advocacy from within and from outside health professions, 6–9
Institute for Health Care Improvement (IHI) (case study), 24–25
Institute of Medicine, 14
Institute on Medicine as a Profession Program (IMAP), 9
Insurance, as unmet legal needs, 84–85, 94
Internet-based continuing medical education (CME), 19
Interviews and media campaign
  basics, 72
  preparing for, 71–72
  and television, 73
IRS 990-PFs tax documents, 175

Jackson v. Motel 6 Multipurpose, Inc., 1997, 110
Jargon and acronyms, avoidance of, 72–73
Joint guardianship proceeding, 92
Josiah Macy Foundation, 9
Journal of the American Medical Association (JAMA), 4
Justhealth.info, 93

KLAY V. HUMANA, INC., 115–119
Knowledge, for advocacy training, 23
Knowledge/skill transfer, 20

Lawhelp.org, 93
Lead counsel, appointment of, 111
Learning advocacy, 16–17
  putting into practice, 21–25
Learning in context, 20
Learning in the workplace, 20
Legal advocacy, 82

Legal help, referring patients to, 93, 94–97
Legal status, as unmet legal needs, 91, 96
Legislative advocacy, 37, 51
  advancing a cause, 56–57
  bill, passing, 54
  bill becoming law, 52–56
  communicate a message, 57–60
  constituent, 59
  expert speakers, 58
  face time, 58
  Federal Senators, 53
  first reading, 54
  Nebraska's Legislature, 52
  relationship building, 56, 57
  second reading, 54
  State Children's Health Insurance Program (SCHIP) (case study), 61–63
  third reading, 54
  town hall meetings, 58–59
  tracking legislation, 59–60
  using media for, 60–61
  voice vote, 54
Legislative aides, 138
Legislative offices, staff members in, 66
Legislative policy instrument, 41
Letters to the editor, 73–74
Liaison Committee on Medical Education, 2010 report of, 8
Litigation, 30
"The Lived Experience of Becoming an Occupational Therapist," 6
Lobbyists, 44

Media, 65, 66–67
  campaign, 65
  connecting people with, 69
  contact list, 70–71
  crafting the message, 68
  digital realm, 76
  earned media versus paid media, 68–69
  exposure, 65
  "Healthy Minds, Healthy Lives" campaign (case study), 78–79
  interview
    basics, 72

preparing for, 71–72
and television, 73
jargon and acronyms, avoidance of, 72–73
knowing the media, 69
letters to the editor, 73–74
op-eds, 74–75
opportunities, 75–76
social media, 76–78
starting working with, 67
Media case study, 194–196
Media events, 42
Medical–legal partnerships (MLPs), 2, 82, 97
outcomes, 98–99
Medication errors, 124–125
MIND Institute, development of, 152–153
Multiple states' legislation, 60

National Association of Immigration Judges (NAIJ), 129
National Center for Medical–Legal Partnership (NCMLP), 2, 98
National giving, 158, 159
National Subclass, 116
Nebraska's Legislature, 52
New York Times, 4
Non-profit websites, 175
Notice and opt-out class, 112–113
Numerosity analysis, 107–108
Nurses
  medication administration, 124
  shortage of, 137–138

Observation, 20
Oil Pollution Act of 1990, 33
Oklahoma Alliance on Health or Tobacco, 184
Oklahoma Fit Kids Alliance, 190
Oklahoma legislature, 182
Oklahoma Restaurant Association, 187
Online ads, 68
OntracK Campaign, 183
Op-eds, 74–75
Open Congress, 59

Paid media, earned media versus, 68–69
Parent/family organizations as partners, 144–145
Autism Society of America (ASA) (case study), 145–146
Personal and family stability
  as unmet legal needs, 91–92, 96–97
Petition for homestead, 93
Philanthropy, 174
  partnership in, 175
Plaintiffs, class actions and, 107
Policy advocacy, 29–30
Policy change, goals of, 36
Policy evaluation, 45
Policy implementation and evaluation, 45
Policy tools/instruments, 36–37
Political advocacy process, 29
  evaluating challenges to public health goal, 31
  assessing voter awareness of problem, 32
  causation of problem, 31
  current policy environment, 31–32
  defining the problem, 31
  evidence-based policy design, 34
  designing the new policy, 36–39
  using scientific research in advocacy, 34–36
  executing the strategic plan, 41
  drafting the policy instrument, 41
  getting and keeping the public on your side, 41–43
  identifying potential policymaker champions, 41
  launching the campaign, 43
  swaying the policymakers, 43–45
  policy implementation and evaluation, 45
  strategic plan, 39
  policy venue, 39–40
  timetable for action, 39
  understanding and combating the opposition, 40
  supporting organizations, alliance of, 32
  building an advocacy alliance, 32–34
  effective alliance infrastructure, 34
Political advocates, 30

Positive impact, demonstrating, 177
Practice of advocacy, leveraging research findings in, 121
  analytic method, selecting, 129–130
  findings, presentation of, 130–131
  funding for, 125–127
  in health policy, 138–139
  nursing workforce, expanding (case study), 134–138
  for patient care, 136–138
  problem, identifying, 123–125
  quantitative study, descriptive findings from, 135–136
  research, reasons for, 122
  research questions, developing, 127–129
  school counselors, qualitative method study of (case study), 132–133
Predominance standard, 110
Presentation of research findings, 130–131
Press conferences, 42
Press releases, 42
PRIME-US, 7
Prior knowledge
  activation of, 20
  linking newly learned skills to, 23
Private donors, 173–175
Promotion of advocacy, from within and from outside health professions, 6–9
Public health goal, evaluating challenges to, 31
  assessing voter awareness of problem, 32
  causation of problem, 31
  current policy environment, 31–32
  defining the problem, 31
Public policy, 29
Public policy advocacy, 29

Qualitative Health Research, 129
Qualitative research, methods for, 129–130

Racketeer Influenced and Corrupt Organization (RICO), 115
Relationship building, 56, 57
Reporters, contacts with, 71
Representative, meeting with, 58
Research case study, 197–200
Research findings, presentation of, 122, 130–131
Research method, selection of, 129–130
Research questions, developing, 127–129
Restaurant Association bill, 188, 189
Retainer agreement, 111
Rimland, Bernard, 145
Robert Wood Johnson Foundation (RWJF), 134
Role plays, 23

Safety of patients, identifying, 124
SB1553, 185
SB696, 186
Scale item surveys, 130
Secondary data analyses, 130
Second reading, 54
Self-direction, 20
Self-efficacy, 20
Service learning, 8
Shaywitz, David, 3
Sherman Act, 115
SJR36, 183
Skill gap, of advocacy, 15–16
"Slippery slope" effect, 40
Smoke-free legislation, in Oklahoma, 185
"Socially responsible and idealistic" physicians, 7
Social media, 76–78
State Business and Consumer Protection Laws, 115
State Children's Health Insurance Program (SCHIP) (case study), 61–63
State legislative process, 56
State legislative tracking, 60
Statutes related to business, 115
Stewardship, 171, 175
Stoneridge Inv. Partners, *LLC v. Scientific-Atlanta*, 2008, 106
Strategic plan, 39
  executing, 41
  drafting the policy instrument, 41
  getting and keeping the public on your side, 41–43

identifying potential policymaker champions, 41
launching the campaign, 43
swaying the policymakers, 43–45
policy venue, 39–40
timetable for action, 39
understanding and combating the opposition, 40
Strong alliance leadership, 33
Supporting organizations,
alliance of, 32
building an advocacy alliance, 32–34
effective alliance infrastructure, 34
System changes, advocating for, 99–101
Systems-based practice (SBP), 15

Television, media training for, 73
Third reading, 54
THOMAS, 59
Tobacco control in Oklahoma, 182
Tobacco-Free Oklahoma Coalition, 182
Tobacco Use Prevention and Cessation Revolving Fund, 183
Town hall meetings, 58–59
Tracking legislation, 59–60
Traditional media advertising, 68
Transitional care, model of, 126
Twitter, 77
Typicality, 108–110

Undergraduate medical education (UME), 15
Unger v. Amedisys Inc., 2005, 110
Unmet legal needs
education, 87–89, 95
employment, 89–90, 96
housing, 85–87, 95
identifying, 82
income, 83–84, 94
insurance, 84–85, 94
legal status, 91, 96
medical–legal partnerships, 97
outcomes, 98–99
personal and family stability, 91–92, 96–97
planning for advanced care, 92–93, 97
referring patients to legal help, 93, 94–97
system changes, advocating for, 99–101
U.S. health care system, 13

Voice vote, 54
Volunteers in fundraising, 172–173
Voter awareness of problem, assessing, 32

Web-based continuing medical education (CME), 19

Made in the USA
Lexington, KY
25 August 2017